Denial to Acceptance

Denial to Acceptance

From a breast cancer season to gratefulness

Cynthia Langdon

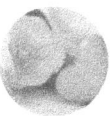

Cynthia Langdon

Disclaimer

The information contained in this book is for general information purposes only. The information is provided by Cynthia Langdon, and while we endeavour to keep the information up to date and correct. I make no representations or warranties of any kind, expressed or implied, about the completeness, accuracy, reliability, suitability, or availability with respect to this publication or the information, products, services, or related graphics contained in this publication for any purpose. Any reliance you place on such information is therefore strictly at your own risk. In no event, will we be liable for any loss or damage, including, without limitation, indirect or consequential loss or damage. Or any loss or damage whatsoever arising from loss of data or profits, arising out of, or in connection with, the use of this publication. Through this publication, you are able to link to other resources and contacts which are not under the control of Cynthia Langdon. We have no control over the nature, content, and availability of those responsible for their management, operation, or function. The inclusion of any links does not necessarily imply a recommendation or endorse the views expressed within them. At the time of writing, every effort was made to keep the information in this publication current. However, Cynthia Langdon takes no responsibility for, and will not be liable for, information being out of date or unavailable, due to technical or any other issue beyond our control.

Contact Cynthia Langdon at: cynthialangdonbook@gmail.com

Copyright Year: November 2021, First edition
Copyright Notice: Published by Cynthia Langdon. All rights reserved. No part of this book may be reproduced in any form or by any means whatsoever, unless where permission is granted by Cynthia Langdon.

Results in this copyright notice:

© 2021 Cynthia Langdon. All rights reserved

ISBN: 978-1-4717-0708-7

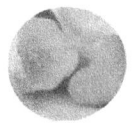

Denial to Acceptance

From a breast cancer season to gratefulness

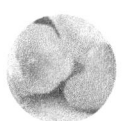

Cynthia Langdon

FOR

Supporting the fighters

Admiring the survivors

Honouring the taken:

My Mum -Verona Sandy Langdon

Jodie Fitzgerald

Stacey White

Janine Ann Brook

And never ever giving up HOPE

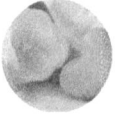

Denial to Acceptance

Table of Contents

About the Author 6
Foreword 8
Chapter 1 - My Childhood Days 11
Chapter 2 - Diagnosis and Procedures 31
Chapter 3 - Treatment 51
Chapter 4 - Recovery 72
Chapter 5 - Lifestyle Changes Days 85
Chapter 6 - Reflections 103
Chapter 7 - A New Life 119
Chapter 8 - Men and Breast Cancer 123
Chapter 9 - Facts and More Information 128
Chapter 10 - I *Hope* One Day: A Cure for Breast Cancer 139
Chapter 11 - My Experience on Surviving 143
Chapter 12 - My Special Messages to You 152
Preface 158
Acknowledgements 159
Recognition 161

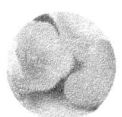

About the Author

Born and raised in East London, to Grenadian parents Verona and Norris. The youngest of four siblings, sister, aunty, glamourous great aunty, godmother, relative, friend. With a background in banking, Cynthia eventually became a civil servant, then entrepreneur by operating her own travel business. She believes in personal growth by expanding and being responsible for her self-development, self-care, knowledge and improving her personal skills in all areas of her life. Cynthia is a risk-taker and loves challenges.

Introduction

I had a dream that I would become a TV/Radio presenter, hosting my own health and wellbeing lifestyle show. My goal was achieved, and I managed to get a monthly slot on *LUV316*, an online radio station owned by my cousin Lucas Langdon, who is no longer with us. I hosted my first show three days after I received the news of the breast cancer diagnosis, and still managed to host a further show, before I was forced to take time off to prepare for the sudden and unexpected changes in my life. Along the way, I participated in several Breast Cancer awareness campaigns and in September 2016, I participated in the Breast Cancer Now (previously Breast Cancer Care) *"Here from Day 1"* campaign and in October 2016, I

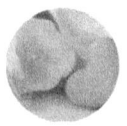

was one of the model ambassadors at the Breast Cancer Now's Annual Gala and Fashion Show event.

Prior to the diagnosis, I was part of a team who organised and hosted events around public health and wellness. With the support of our chosen charity organisations, our aim was to provide information to the community, raising awareness and understanding of many health issues and concerns. To name a few, we organised events in support of Prostate Cancer, Lupus, Sickle Cell, Stroke, and Heart health. I was super proud of being a part of these important events, contributing to raising awareness whilst helping the community.

I decided to write this book because my story mattered, and it needed to be told.

Not only was it very therapeutic, I also learned about parts of my past, which I assumed were buried. Writing this book allowed me to connect with others who have gone through the same experiences. My book is about sharing my secrets of survival and offering support to those who may have been faced with a breast cancer diagnosis, including families, friends and relatives of loved ones. Most importantly, helping to raise awareness and prevention of this disease, giving people HOPE!

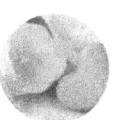

Foreword

It is my absolute pleasure to write the foreword to this wonderfully inspiring and informative book. I am an ex-professional footballer, born in Forest Gate and brought up in Upton Park (yes, West Ham United Football Club territory). The majority of my playing career was at Tottenham Hotspur Football Club and whilst there, I was fortunate enough to have been involved in three FA Cup Finals and a UEFA Cup Final, winning three out of the four. I finished my playing days with short spells at West Ham and Brentford, before returning to Tottenham, to embark on various coaching roles. I was also fortunate to represent the Republic of Ireland, over a ten-year period, playing in Euro '88 and World Cup '90, respectively. Eventually, I ended up at Newcastle United, as a coach and soon became the manager. It was from here my managerial career actually started, and that journey saw me run Birmingham City, Norwich, Brighton & Hove Albion, and Nottingham Forest football clubs too.

It was Cynthia's brother - Clarence - who I first met since we both represented the Borough of Newham at football, so I knew about Cynthia long before we really met. I'm not exactly sure when that was, since we went to different schools, a stone's throw away from each other; I attended St Bonaventure while Cynthia went to St

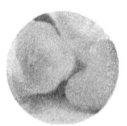

Denial to Acceptance

Angela's. There was a lot of mixing between the two schools, some official and some not, but what I can say is that she was as bubbly, chatty and engaging then, as she is today!

It was in my late teens when I got to know Cynthia, since our meetings were predominantly through her friends and family, who I also got to know. However, eventually, as adults we got to chat regularly, whenever we met on the train and as she headed to work. I think most of us can relate to her work ethic too, being brought up in a working-class area, and families that stressed the importance of working.

In my profession, I'm used to seeing players endure bad injuries, some of which can be career-threatening or ending. The mental and physical anguish, connected with their rehabilitation, is challenging enough and yet, nothing can be compared to somebody fighting cancer and what they go through. Fortunately, Cynthia and I have the same cultural support network, and we can and do lean on when we need to. Seeing her go through this journey made me realise that, sometimes having them, was enough or sometimes, not at all.

Still, I am privileged to be part of the close-knit group of people, who experienced Cynthia's journey. Especially, to see her share how she navigated each chapter and stage of her fight. Here, in this book,

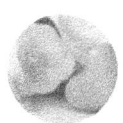

she refers to those people and organisations that supplemented that network. As someone who has a lot of women within a big family, I have learned so much about breast cancer, and the emotions associated with it. In this book, that touches us all.

Cynthia has always been family oriented and knows the value of having good friends, and that was always obvious to everyone around her, and about her. Her personality, motivation and drive, blossomed in this environment, helping her with her rehabilitation and recovery, and beyond. As the years rolled by, Cynthia has not changed. She holds onto those values and qualities that are important to her. Those, which have helped her to overcome.

This book is about a down-to-earth lady, sharing her highs and lows, emotions and education, and also finding herself through the mental, physical and spiritual processes, and her coping mechanisms.

Chris Hughton
Ex-Professional Football Player
Ex-Professional Football Club Manager

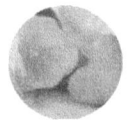

Chapter 1 - My Childhood Days

Everyone enters the world as a baby, growing through a phase of growth called childhood. Childhood is a part of life that can create beautiful memories.

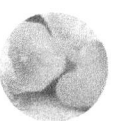

Cynthia Langdon

Mum and Dad

My childhood days were content. I came from a happy, respectful family home, where I lived with my Mum – Verona, Dad – Norris, my siblings – Clarence and Gloria. An elder sibling – Edith, lived in the Caribbean, on the beautiful island of *"sugar and spice" Grenada*. She was the lucky one, living in the sunshine with our grandmother, my Mum's mum. I was the youngest. My mother was a nurse, who worked extremely hard to keep her family together, making sure we always had food on the table and clothes on our backs. We were always shown love and care.

Dad was a carpenter, though you would never believe that. He worked on a building site and would go to work in a three-piece suit and tie, carrying a briefcase that contained his sandwiches. He loved his sweet scent of aftershave, and it was when he reached work where he would put on his overalls.

In the early 1980s, Mum was diagnosed with breast cancer. I was in my early 20s, and her treatment involved mastectomy and radiotherapy. Mum had one breast removed, and I believe, five years later, she had the other breast removed, for precautionary reasons. I remember going to the London Hospital in Whitechapel, for appointments with her. Back then, I never really knew too much

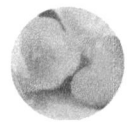

about breast cancer. Why did it happen? How one got it, the treatment and so on. To be honest, I didn't even realise it was a life-threatening disease. Yet, she was always full of spirit and upbeat, and if she was low during those times, she never showed it, or I never noticed. But then, my Mum always loved to laugh, even when she was sad.

Mum lived with this disease for many years, and on 6th September 1995, she was sadly taken away from us. Mum had gone to Grenada for a six-month break and to attend my elder sister's wedding. But it was cut short, because she started to feel unwell and returned sooner than expected. She was feeling aches and pains, especially around her hips, had a loss of appetite and appeared to lose weight. She appeared to be getting shorter in height although she was not a tall lady. There were days when she could not leave her bed, and this was hard. Mum, and her children, had no idea what was going on with her illness at this stage. In appointments with Mum's doctor and hospital consultants, they informed us that Mum suffered with osteoporosis and brittle bones; a bone disease that occurs when the body loses too much bone, making too little bone or both. As a result, bones become weak and could break from a fall. At this time, even though mum had two mastectomy surgeries and radiotherapy

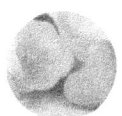

treatments, we had no idea the reason for her osteoporosis was due to the cancer recurring and spreading to her bones!

I had visited Mum's doctor to arrange for a home visit, because Mum was unable to attend the surgery. Her doctor said the cancer had spread to her bones. This left me in utter disbelief, wounded and shocked.

So, when he told me the reason for her aches and pains and that they were due to the cancer returning and spreading to her bones, it hit like a strong earthquake. *What on earth is he talking about?* Nobody – the family and Mum included – realised the cancer would return, let alone spread to her bones. I remember Mum saying on more than one occasion: *"I'm sure the cancer has returned"*.

Six weeks to the date of being told of her diagnosis, Mum passed away! I was 35 years of age, and no one expects to lose a parent. I was not prepared. Six months prior to Mum's death, my cousin, and best friend Laureen Mitchell, also passed away. Laureen and I enjoyed raving together. She loved her soul music, loved to dance, kept fit and healthy, and was always helpful and supportive to everyone who came in contact with her. We were always enjoying ourselves, at some event or the other. Laureen's death was the very first close relative death I had experienced, and it was her death that

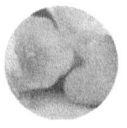

brought everything to a halt. Then it was Mum passing, six months later.

I was confused, anxious, numb and angry, and I felt my life was falling apart. Mum's passing did not sink in. I did not know how to grieve, and on the outside, I pretended I was fine but struggled to accept that she was gone on the inside. I threw myself back into work three weeks after Mum was gone. One day, on my way to work, I met one of the nurses who worked with Mum. She asked how I was feeling and said it was time for me to move on. I was surprised by her statement! My Mother and I shared a special bond, and I expected her to be with me forever. I lost a part of me, my greatest advocate and did not realise there was a cut-off time to move on from the loss of a mother, father, relative, friend. However, I tried to move on with my life, but I was going through several emotions and was not being true to myself, ending up suffering with anxiety. This resulted in me being signed off from work for 3 months. I was working at Barclays Bank, in Liverpool Street, at the time.

After Mum died, I did not know what the rest of my life had in store for me. A lot of it was a blur in the beginning. The person who carried me for nine months and brought me into the world was no longer here. I felt a part of me was missing. It was one of the toughest and

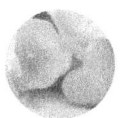

painful things I had to deal with. Not everybody is ever interested in everything you do or as proud as your mother.

I eventually found peace and healing by creating *a memory box* with special Birthday/Christmas cards and beautiful pictures of Mum laughing, dancing and enjoying herself. The days I felt low, I would open the box, and it would always give me a real ray of sunshine -

Verona's Ray of Sunshine. Mother is always the beginning - she is how things begin. Mum was the hub of family life and I know that her dream was to see her children grow to be happy and successful.

Dad contracted lung cancer and passed away in June 2004.

Mum and Dad were separated, and I was uncertain as to why. He was not around much when Mum had her second mastectomy, but when she felt poorly, he visited often. Dad was a person who loved life, adored partying, and I think that was where I got my party moves. When we were growing up, he was strict with me and I was always being told off, not allowed to do this, go there, be home at a certain time and needed to give two weeks' notice whenever I wanted to go out – really! I was seventeen or eighteen years of age, working, earning a good salary and had a decent boyfriend.

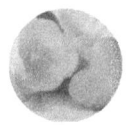

Denial to Acceptance

I remember when I first introduced my Dad to my first boyfriend, Keith, and the first thing he said:

"What's your intention?"

I could have sunk into a hole. Dad hadn't even greeted him: *good morning or afternoon, I'm pleased to meet you!* But Keith held his own and said he intended to look after me - and he did for five years.

I always challenged my Dad and was fearful, whenever he raised his voice and to this day, I dislike raised voices or being shouted at. When my Dad shouted, I would tremble, but that did not stop me disagreeing with him. Our cat, Sooty, was scared of my Dad's raised voice too and would run and hide under the dining room table, when he saw Dad enter the family home. Still, Dad never knew I used to wait for him to leave home, so that I could sneak out to meet my friends. On the weekends, my friend Jeanne and I always had some place to go, starting from Thursday night. It was a great time of fun and laughter, and I was truly grateful for those days. Looking back, I really don't know where the energy came from.

One thing I did not understand about my Dad was that he was always disciplining me about going out when he was always out himself, whether at bingo, the pub, some party like a boat party. Yes, you guessed it – Dad was a right raver, and his nickname was *Saga Man*.

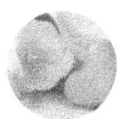

After Mum passed, and years later, Dad remarried and I did not see much of him then. My brother kept in regular contact and told me of his illness. I visited him regularly. Dad had been a smoker and those around him were smokers too and, unfortunately, he contracted lung cancer. I was sad when he passed. I remember visiting him at the chapel of rest and couldn't even bring myself to view his body. I don't know why. Anyway, wherever he was, I was sure he was having a great time. I loved both my parents, and thank them for creating me into the strong, bold, powerful, fearless and prosperous person I am today.

St Angela's Ursuline Convent School

Mum sent me to St Angela's Ursuline Convent School in Forest Gate and my brother to a mixed school in Manor Park, Little Ilford. My cousins – Yvonne and Laureen, also attended the convent, which was why Mum wanted me to go there. Since we lived outside the catchment area, it was a challenge to get in. I was only accepted because my cousins attended, and I attended Saturday School.

You would think that with me attending a convent school, I would be an angel, but far from it. I often played truant, and I was once sent home by Sister Mark, the Head Teacher, because I went to school without wearing any socks. In the early 70s the summers were

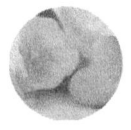

scorchers, and so I decided I was going to wear a summer dress with my Jesus Creepers sandals, without socks.

These were also worn by nuns and monks at the school and in assembly that morning, Sister Mark called me out in front of the entire student body. I was told to go home and not return until I was wearing socks. Mum was very displeased. I would also roll up my skirt, because it reached my ankles and my blazer's arms, since they covered my hands. That was how Mum bought them. I got told off for rolling up my skirt, and it was funny because I always made the back longer than the front. In the end, I gave up and wore it as an ankle skirt and did not attempt to make it into a mini.

One day in a cookery class, I did not like what we needed to prepare. So, after lunch, I escaped and went to my friend's house. We played music, danced and laughed, but the school contacted Mum and told her I was missing. Imagine, a parent of that generation, hearing from a teacher that their child was missing from school; especially a convent school. Ouch! Anyway, after my interaction with Mum, let's just say, I never missed school again; even when I suffered bad abdominal pains, asthma or hay-fever. To make that day worse, Mum also learned from my brother's school that he too was also missing

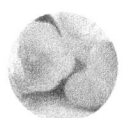

that afternoon. Not that we planned it but suffice to say, our punishments made sure we did not do it again.

I was always caught laughing and in Math's class, Sister Beatrice would always send me to stand outside by the classroom door, on top of getting detention. I admit Math's was not one of my stronger subjects since I was rarely in the classroom and what Sister Beatrice never realised was my schoolmates were chatting behind her back. Yet, whenever she turned around, I was the one she caught laughing. Naturally, I would never snitch on my schoolmates. However, by the end of the term when my school report was done, it always said: *"Cynthia is a good worker, but easily distracted"*.

Friendships

My childhood was great. I love and cherish the memories. I had great classmates and forty plus years today are still great friends – Pam, Cheryl, Bridget, Frances, Gloria Imbert, Joanne, Audrey, Justina, Barbara, Sonia and Vivienne. I was fortunate to have these ladies in my life during this breast cancer season. They were in shock when they learned of the breast cancer diagnosis but, supported me one hundred percent. Even though they had their own lives to live, they found time to send me messages, make a phone call, or visit when appropriate. I was blessed with kindness.

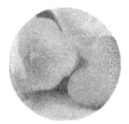

Career and My Young Adult Life

After leaving school, I attended East Ham Technical College, where I studied a secretarial course. After one year, I applied for a job and began in the typing pool at the Department for Health and Social Security (DHSS) as it was known, and now the Department for Work and Pensions (DWP). About a year and a half later, I applied to work at an oil company in the City and then moved to a job at Barclays Bank also in the City. This was where I started as a shorthand and audio typist and worked my way up to a secretary/personal assistant. Eventually, I was offered voluntary redundancy due to organisational restructuring and after sixteen years I left. Back then, moving from one job to the next was easier than it was now and the experience I gained, I was grateful for.

My life was changing. I was growing up. I was earning a good salary and began to travel and explore the world, and from the age of twenty-one, I began to play netball competitively with an unbeatable netball team called *Caribbean International*, making lifelong friends along the way.

In addition to my extracurricular activities, I was only interested in working, earning, buying my own clothes, shoes, handbags, and travelling. Since, I figured life was about enjoying oneself and having

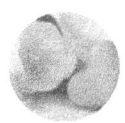

fun. After all, the time before Mum passed, I was still living at home and my sole responsibility was giving her grocery money. I had no other commitments. Those early years of my life were great. No pressure or stress, and how I wished my life could always be like that.

There was one goal I had and that was by the time I was twenty-five years of age, I wanted to be married with two children. After all, that was what growing up meant – leave school, go to college, begin work, meet your soulmate, get engaged, buy your dream home, get married, and start a family. Well…that did not happen. Life was moving fast, and I was living my best life. Then I met Lloyd Wilson. On reflection, Lloyd – who has now passed, wanted to settle down, but I was not ready. I realised that at my age I was still young and there was still so much I wanted to do for myself before I settled down. I wanted to have fun, explore the world, and not have a family yet. At times, though, I wondered what my life would have been like if I had accepted his proposal.

My Sibling, his Friends, and *Jah Conqueror Sound System*

When I look back on my childhood, I was always working on some project, reading or listening to music. Our home was always warm and welcoming, and in those days my brother operated a sound

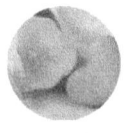

system with his friends. *My brothers from another mother* – Paul, Stanley, Peter, Quinn, Lewis, Michael, Cliff, and Anthony built their sound system in Mum's back garden. They built big, heavy black boxes and would play "choons". Their sound was called Jah *Conqueror Sound System*. Those were great times.

Even though, now older and moved in different directions, we are still great friends to this day. They were also very supportive of me, during my breast cancer season.

My brother and I grew up in Manor Park with Peter and Quinn and their sister Donna. In our youth days, Donna and I were the only supporting young ladies that followed their sound system to their gigs when they regularly played at East Ham Town Hall and house parties. Donna and I had the privilege of getting into these gigs for free and because they were our brothers, they were very protective of us. On occasions, we helped carry the record box.

Changes in the Family Home

Eventually, our family home changed. My brother and his wife Sandra purchased a property. They also had Leona, their daughter, now married and a mother of two gorgeous children: my great niece Saniya, and great nephew, Shaylen. Both keep me on my toes. My

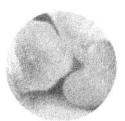

sister Gloria was married and started her new life with her husband, and I purchased my very first flat in Leyton.

It was when I left the family home that I believe I started to experience severe abdominal aches and pains. Once, my doctor told me I would never have children (because I had signs of abnormal cell growths) and to be honest, in my early twenties, I was not overly concerned since I was having fun exploring the world. So, I accepted what he told me without question. At the time, I was uncertain whether I was carrying any resentfulness or disappointment and never questioned whether I was really worried I would be unable to have children and be a mum. The question everyone asked themselves would be: *why me?*

But, to my surprise, I was able to conceive. I was in total shock when it was confirmed, and I struggled with this, since I feared losing my child. *"Was this why my baby died, or was it because of the abnormal cell growths known as fibroids?"* A story for another time. However, my main ambition was about living the societal dream – school, college, work, soul mate, house, marriage, family and watching the grandkids grow up! I was really looking forward to what I had planned for my life. But as I now know, plans and your life can change…in the blink of an eye.

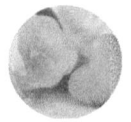

The Strain and Stress of Relationships

In life, I have learnt that we make plans for our lives, but, situations, circumstances, and misfortunes can get in the way at any time. We lose friends and family along our life's journey or at times, they detach themselves from us, to become strangers. I experienced this with my immediate family. It was a pretty emotional and depressing time of my life. Relationships became strained, and it was difficult for anyone to be their true self. The tension caused me to be unsettled mentally, emotionally, spiritually, and ultimately physically. The resulting signs manifested themselves in me since I contracted my illness. Naturally and in hindsight, I was only aware of how much this episode played a big role in my life when I got the chance to go through my life-changing experience. Mum had always taught me to be kind. I learnt that we cannot control the behaviour, attitude or actions of others. We can only control ourselves.

Life before My Diagnosis

In 2008, I was shocked to notice a tiny, pea-size lump on my right breast, just above my nipple. It was painless but firm and *scared out of my wits* was an understatement. My mum had breast cancer, leaving this world on 6th September 1995 and those memories of her

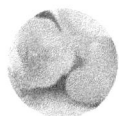

came flooding back. At the time, I thought, *"Please do not tell me that I may now have breast cancer too?"*

Panicking, I immediately rang my GP and made an emergency appointment. I did not tell anyone about this, since I did not want to unnecessarily burden anyone. Trust me that was hard to do, because whenever I had a simple ache, pain, spot, or pimple on my face, everyone knew about it. I was seen by my GP within a week, and she referred me to the hospital for a mammogram or breast screening and biopsy. Within two weeks of seeing my GP, I was seen at the hospital.

This was one of the most painful days of my life and waiting for the results of both the mammogram and biopsy was an absolute nightmare. However, I went on with my daily life until I received them. It was extremely difficult keeping my composure during that time. Two weeks after visiting the hospital I received an appointment letter in the post, to attend for the results.

When the results came, I remember walking into the hospital in complete fear. I was welling up and my mind worked overtime. *What am I going to do? How will I survive having breast cancer? Will I need breast reconstruction? How was I going to break the news to my family and friends?*

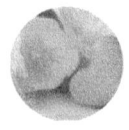

Denial to Acceptance

Sitting in the hospital waiting area, my name was called, and I jumped from my seat, hailing: *Yes, that's me.* A nurse escorted me to the consultant's room, and I walked in with a smile, and said good morning.

The consultant introduced himself: *"Good morning, Miss Langdon, we have your results".*

My palms were sweating and I was tearing up. My entire body shook, I was a nervous wreck.

"We have your results", he repeated, *"you have a benign tumour called Fibroadenoma."* (Or not cancerous).

"Sorry", I said, *"what is this?"*

Since I couldn't even pronounce it. He explained that it was a non-cancerous breast lump but because it was small, they did not need to do anything. However, he said that these kinds of lumps could grow over the years and become unsightly and if that happened, I would need to return to have it removed. *WOW!!* I was so excited that I shook his hand, thanking him and skipping out of the room and out of the hospital; smiling like a Cheshire cat. *I don't have breast cancer, yippee. Thank you, Lord.* When I got home, I Googled

Fibroadenoma to learn about it and soon continued with my life as normal.

Find out about fibroadenoma (breastcancernow.org)

It was during September to December 2013 when I noticed a change in my body. A strong, regular pain occurred from my right arm; however, I assumed it was muscular and came from lifting weights. I did not think it could be connected to breast cancer. There were moments of dizziness and jaw ache on my right side, and I was generally feeling unwell. Although I couldn't understand why this was happening, I still carried on with my daily routine. I also noticed how the same lump above my nipple started to grow and felt rubbery and changed colour. I usually examined myself and, even more so, with the sudden change in my breast's appearance. Although I felt at ease, I couldn't feel or see any further lumps around my breast and nipple areas. But I remember Mauray saying to me that I needed to get the lump checked as it could be cancer. I thought, *"don't be silly"* and shrugged off the word, believing that it was just the fibroadenoma growing back, as the consultant said it could, over the years.

At this stage, I was not scared. However, I made an appointment to see my GP. She arranged for me to have a full health check – blood,

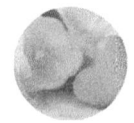

cholesterol, eye, ear, kidney, urine, and diabetes. All the results came back fine. But on examining the lump, I was told that it looked like an infection and was given antibiotics for seven days. I started to feel better, the lump did not improve nor was it painful, but it did begin to increase in size. I made a further appointment to see my GP and asked to be referred to the hospital for further checks. Even then, I still was not concerned that it could be cancerous. I was sure it was the fibroadenoma that had grown, and now it was time to have it removed. On the 18th December 2013, I had a further mammogram and biopsy.

This was painful, but I was sure the results would return negative, and arrangements would be made to have the lump removed. I also visited my dentist because although I was not experiencing any toothache, I was experiencing jaw ache. After being examined, my dentist asked if I was experiencing any form of stress because she noticed I was grinding my teeth; a symptom of stress. At the time, I was not worried about anything in particular nor was I aware, until my dentist pointed it out. My dentist encouraged me to return to my GP for a further full and thorough check-up.

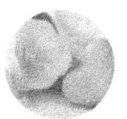

Upon reflection, there were events in my life at the time that I was anxious about, which I avoided. I did not realise that by being this way it would have a serious effect on my body.

Chapter 2 - Diagnosis and Procedures

- Chemotherapy Surgery
- Radiotherapy
- Psychotherapy

"In the blink of an eye, my whole life changed"

A journey of overcoming isolation, fear, mental and physical emotions, to embracing and living a most beautiful life, you'd never believe that cancer can and would be a personal part of you.

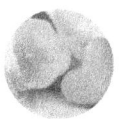

The week after Christmas 2013, I received a telephone call from the hospital asking if I could attend on 7th January 2014. It was a cold wintry evening and I went to King George's Hospital for the appointment. There was no need to ask anyone to come with me because I was not expecting to hear any sad news, and plus it was a dark and bleak evening. I felt they were going to tell me about the results from the mammogram and biopsy were negative and arrangements would be made to have the fibroadenoma removed. I was so wrong.

My appointment was scheduled for 7pm and I arrived about ten minutes early. The waiting room was pretty quiet. I went up to the receptionist's desk to check in and was asked to wait to be called by the consultant. I happily read my book whilst I waited. It was 7.50pm when I heard my name called by a nurse and she took me to the consultant's room. The consultant was sitting behind a desk, said good evening and introduced himself as Mr Ojo. I said good evening to Mr Ojo, and he asked me to take a seat. He then went on to say that the results from my biopsy had returned and that I had breast cancer.

"Excuse me," I said, *"are you having a laugh?"*

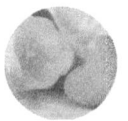

Denial to Acceptance

I started laughing and thought, *"What did he just say?"* He then went on to say we must act quickly because it had spread to my lymph nodes. Now he was really putting the shivers up my spine. *"What on earth are you talking about"?* I silently asked.

He went on to say that you will start by having chemotherapy for six months, followed by a lumpectomy to remove the lump, then radiotherapy and Herceptin treatments. *"What on earth are you talking about?"* I thought.

I told him I couldn't have breast cancer because I would be starting my radio lifestyle show on Saturday. I couldn't have anything disrupting my plans. But my situation showed me that life could change in a blink of an eye – plans or no plans!

I was in total shock, disbelief and denial, and started shaking and crying. Thoughts of my mum came flooding back. I remember the nurse holding my hand, and handing me some breast cancer booklets and leaflets, but I kept thinking: *"Oh my gosh, who will look after me?"* I was not scared of the inevitability of death, but I feared suffering and the thought of having chemotherapy scared me. Especially, since I witnessed some of my loved ones go through it, the overwhelming pain, loss of weight and the inability to help

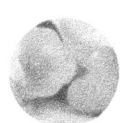

themselves. I was thinking, I really did not want to go through this. I couldn't go through the pain and torture.

I began to blame myself, wondering what I had done wrong, or what could I have done differently to prevent this happening? OK, I loved the odd glass of red wine and a Bacardi and coke on occasions. I ate well and very rarely ate sweets, chocolate, biscuits, and cakes. I exercised regularly, had fun and laughter around me, life was good – so *why me*?

One sign and symptom of breast cancer is the aches and pains under the armpit which I was experiencing and maybe through my ignorance, ignored it, unaware that this was actually a symptom. I would like to say to every person reading this, please be aware of the signs and symptoms and **do not** ignore any unusual aches or pain.

I **AM** here to share my story with you – the world, and I hope you will find comfort, inspiration, and motivation in knowing that any illness or misfortune that we face can be overcome. After finding acceptance and doing everything in our power to find peace, joy, happiness, love, and support.

During this time of my life, there were days when I felt isolated, especially when it came to the pain and exhaustion I experienced.

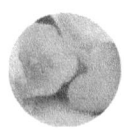

But it was comforting knowing I was not alone. This was not a time for me to be a super heroine! I needed help, and I was willing to ask and receive help.

Okay, I accepted. It is true, I have got a breast cancer diagnosis, but "I don't have to like it or let it define who I am". I knew I had to fight for my life, especially since I was getting all the help and support out there for me. At the age of fifty-four, on 7th January 2014, I was diagnosed with Human Epidermal Growth Receptor 2 (HER2), positive breast cancer that had spread to my lymph nodes. A cancer that has a higher-than-normal level of protein and has the potential to spread to other parts of the body (further information can be found www.breastcancernow.org[1]).

On 22nd January 2014, I met my Clinical Oncologist, Dr. Mary Quigley. She was such a cute and kind lady, and a specialist in treating breast cancer at Queen's Hospital, Romford. The hospital catered well for their patients' visits and offered various things, such as coffee shops, restaurants, convenience stores, a fruit stall, cash machines, baby feeding areas, Wi-Fi, and a special small car park

---

[1] Source: Breast Cancer Now – HER2: https://breastcancernow.org/.../diagnosed-breastcancer/her2

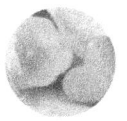

for patients. So, an entire day there could tend to be a comfortable one.

Sandra, my sister-in-law, accompanied me, and we arrived on time. At reception, I gave my name and waited to be called. I had no idea, but soon realised that there was so much information to take in, and I was grateful for Sandra being there with me. Dr Quigley explained the treatment and drugs that would be administered.

At the time, I had no clue what these drugs were. However, I was given an information leaflet explaining how the treatment would be administered and the common side effects. This included infection such as viral and bacterial, hair loss, mouth ulcers, tiredness, nausea, sickness, lack of appetite and mood swings. Other treatments included regular ultrasounds to look at the changes in the breast and bone density scans to look at the conditions of the bones and prevent any risks of weakened bones.

Dr. Quigley went on to explain that after my treatment of six months, I would need surgery to remove the lump on my breast and lymph nodes, followed by a three-week course of radiotherapy treatment. She said I would be given *Anastrozole,* a hormone tablet that was known to help to suppress oestrogen. She stressed that on starting chemotherapy, it would take between seven and ten days to have an

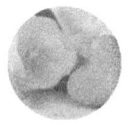

effect on my body. And with all this information bombarding me, I was still in complete shock, doubt and denial. A mixture of emotions of sadness of the unknown. I felt vulnerable because I was not in control. These thoughts came to me:

- *Can I survive the treatment?*
- *Why should I get treatment and I'll die anyway?*
- *I'm going to die? I don't want to*
- *I'm going to lose part of my body*
- *After surgery, will I still be attractive?*
- *This isn't fair*
- *Why was I not protected from this?*
- *This can't be true*
- *Why me?*
- *Then, why not me? I am not different from any other person*
- *What had I done wrong in my life to deserve this?*
- *What could I have done differently?*
- *Was it Genetic? (Mum was diagnosed with breast cancer many years ago).*

I continued to question myself and the Universe. I believed I looked after myself, ate well, and was kind to myself and others. I believed my lifestyle was healthy, and I was in a loving relationship,

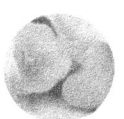

surrounded by caring family and friends. But one thing I did not realise then, was that I was suffering from subconscious stress. There were past events and emotions in my life that were unresolved and unacknowledged. Resulting in worry and sadness, and this I now know played a huge part in my illness.

I questioned why I was being picked on, with so many illnesses. Previously, I had suffered severe menstrual problems at a young age; having fibroids and surgery to remove them, only to return with a vengeance, becoming pregnant but the fibroids interfered with my baby's nutrients, resulting in its death inside me. For two weeks I carried my dead baby because my cervix refused to dilate and, in the end, I had a threatened abortion at six and half months. Now, I have a breast cancer diagnosis. *Really Universe! Really Heavenly Father!*

I was facing yet another incredibly hard, painful, and difficult time in my life. But I knew I also had to choose to stay strong during this time and trust in God, despite the difficulties. I trust God, and I had to continue to pray and have HOPE and JOY that he would give me the Grace I needed to get me through this difficult and painful trial. And yet, the questions continued:

"Did I really have a breast cancer diagnosis?"

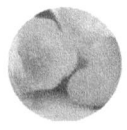

"Was it a mistake?"

"Was this a dream?"

My life was already busy; I couldn't stop to deal with this. I had things to do. I had plans. But the truth was, my plans were put on hold. My life had changed. I had a breast cancer diagnosis. It was not a dream. It was real, and I needed to do my best to come to terms with it. I had to come to terms with the acceptance and adjustment and do everything in my power to heal and recover from this devastating and painful ordeal.

It felt like six months was such a long time, to have poisonous drugs being pumped into my body, especially with life going on. My eldest niece – Leona – was planning her wedding in June of the same year. Yet, just thinking about this allowed me to focus and helped me along the journey. I was so happy I was well enough to attend her wedding since it was my final chemotherapy right after.

Hooray!

My First Chemotherapy Session

Not words one wanted to hear, and certainly not something one wanted to go through.

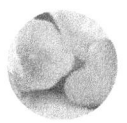

Cynthia Langdon

The night before, I could hardly sleep wondering what to expect. Although I did conduct some research on how to prepare for this first session, I was still very nervous. I remember wearing a sky-blue V-neck jumper and matched this with a blue and white floral scarf, navy leather pencil skirt, and navy velvet boots. I laid out my outfit the night before. I wanted to be prepared by wearing an outfit that was bright and cheerful. I recalled the first day, it was a mild winter morning in early February 2014; the day I had arrived to attend the hospital for my first chemotherapy session. I was anxious because, although I did some research on what to expect, I was still nervous, wondering and questioning myself.

"How long would the treatment be?"

"Would I be sick?"

"Would I have a reaction to the medication?"

"What side effects would I have, immediately after the session?"

"What would the hospital ward look like?"

"Would I be in a room by myself or with other chemotherapy patients"

My cousin, Yvonne Mitchell, collected me from home that morning and took me to my first chemotherapy session. I was relaxed, and we chatted about different things whilst driving to the hospital. When

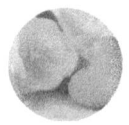

we pulled up at the car park, I had a nervous feeling in my stomach. On entering the hospital, I was warmly greeted by an Oncology nurse for the day. She ushered both Yvonne and I to the Sunflower chemotherapy room. There were some patients on drips lying on beds and some patients sitting on brown leather comfortable couches with drips. The room was actually very bright and colourful with wall-mounted TVs. The Oncology nurse started explaining the process of the chemotherapy drug and how it would be administered. The tears started flowing down my cheeks. I was nervous but both the nurse and my cousin held my hand and comforted me assuring me that everything would be ok. The nurse explained that I would be given intravenous chemotherapy which involves medicine being given slowly from a bag of fluid that is attached with a small tube to one of my veins in the back of my hand.

I completed my first chemotherapy session and felt better than I thought I would and thought Ok, I could probably cope with this once every 3 weeks (*however, little did I know it was the calm before the storm*).

I returned to work the following morning. I was proud of myself for getting through this first chemotherapy session smiling on my way to work and thinking that this was not as bad as I expected. I was happy

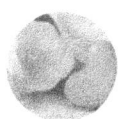

to be at work because I enjoyed my job and being around my colleagues. I loved what I did and was determined that having a cancer diagnosis, or the chemotherapy, would not stop me. I wanted to be normal. I did not want to be known as a cancer patient, and I did not want to put my life on hold. My colleagues knew of my first session and were surprised and concerned to see that I had returned to work the following day. They expected me to be in bed! They were keen to know how I felt and gathered around my desk whilst I gave them an overview of the chemotherapy medicine experience.

That afternoon around 2pm, I received a telephone call from my breast care nurse. She called to find out how I was feeling after the first chemotherapy session. I told her that I was at work and felt fine when I woke up that morning. However, strangely during our conversation I had started developing some symptoms as I became lightheaded and experienced a slight nosebleed, it felt like a hangover (a part of the experience). She demanded I immediately leave work and return home to rest. One of my colleagues offered to drive me home but I had also driven to work and although I felt a little tired, I knew that I would be ok to drive myself back home.

Denial to Acceptance

My colleagues insisted I messaged them as soon as I arrived home and to be honest, I cannot remember if I did at the time because as soon as I arrived home, I just literally threw myself on the bed and dozed off. Though, I was of strong character and would not allow a cancer diagnosis to hold me back, this was a reality check. I finally came to terms with the fact that my condition had put a temporary pause on my life and I needed to start listening to my body; taking responsibility to help myself heal and recover sooner rather than later.

Prior to the breast cancer diagnosis, I had long flowing locks and after 14 years, I felt the need to cut my hair shorter. Mainly, because it started breaking at the forehead and so, it was time to change my image. I decided to cut my hair for charity!

6th September 2013 marked the 18th anniversary of my Mum's end of life to breast cancer and in her memory and support of Breast Cancer Awareness Month. I organised a personal event to raise awareness and funds for *Breast Cancer Now,* by cutting my locks. I was over the moon raising a total of £320. Four months later, I was faced with the devastating news of a breast cancer diagnosis.

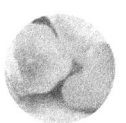

Cynthia Langdon

After My Second Chemotherapy Session

I started losing the rest of my hair. The chemotherapy was beginning to take effect and I needed to deal with it. So, I started wearing head wraps because I wanted to cover my bald head, to keep it warm, and wearing them made me feel comfortable. Head wraps can be glamorous and stylish, and I even learnt how to tie these scarfs into stylish turbans. I accumulated so many head wraps during this season. My closet was filled with big scarves, little scarves, rectangular and square scarves, scarves with prints and scarves without. All the scarves I purchased and wore, during this time of my life, have now been given to charity to help make a difference to someone else's life.

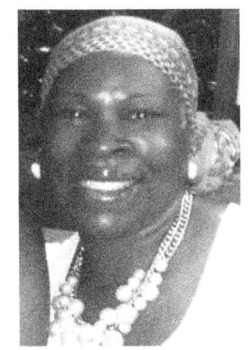

"Being diagnosed with breast cancer is a life-changing moment in a woman's life. It begins a journey of emotional turmoil that will test relationships and individual strength. But, although the future may be uncertain, there is light ahead."

This cancer diagnosis taught me to have a deepened appreciation of life. I wanted to live, be happy with myself, as well as, with everyone and everything around me. I wanted to begin to enjoy my

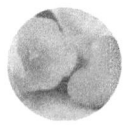

life to the fullest by taking care of my mental and physical wellness and investing time in doing it, travelling whenever given the chance to see new places and meet new people. I wanted to spend time with friends and loved ones instead of wasting time with unimportant things. To do things that gave me pleasure and a sense of satisfaction. I wanted to make the most of my life, despite my circumstances.

I was having chemotherapy every three weeks. Prior to the treatments, I attended hospital two days previously, for a blood test and to be seen by the specialist nurse, in preparation for my chemotherapy drugs. Personally, I was so happy none of my treatments were delayed and just wanted to get it over and done with sooner, rather than later.

The treatment consisted of a nurse inserting a thin, flexible tube or cannula into a vein in my hand. It was painful and uncomfortable, but I grew to tolerate it. I was also given anti-sickness drugs through the tube and rest periods, every three weeks. The first two weeks after treatment I always felt tired; my body ached. At times, I had a loss of appetite, however, I knew that I needed to eat something to maintain my calorie, protein and fluid intake and although fish and chips weren't ideal, it was what I craved at times. I did not feel guilty,

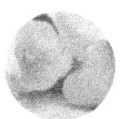

especially when my breast cancer care nurse advised me on occasions, to eat what I liked, to keep my strength up.

The body ache was the unbearable part, and I sometimes felt guilty, staying in bed. But there were days when I lacked energy and enthusiasm. I was exhausted and found it hard to get up in the mornings. I just wanted to stay in bed and couldn't be bothered to do much. This made me feel sad and low. So, I decided to do some research, to find out the cause, it was *cancer fatigue*. I was not just experiencing normal tiredness, but cancer fatigue, which was caused by the cancer and the side effects of chemotherapy. Completely different from normal tiredness. I felt much better and relieved, because it gave me a sense of control, knowing the reason. It was difficult to stay in bed, since I was an active and independent person. However, I knew that to heal and recover I needed to listen to my body.

Tip: *It is important to understand why you are having the drugs. What your body is going through, and why. In my opinion understanding why you are having chemotherapy treatments and what your body is going through is essential for making informed decisions, managing expectations, coping with side effects, and actively participating in*

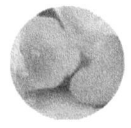

your treatment and recovery process. It empowers you to be an active participant in your care and improves your overall experience throughout the treatment journey.

Supportive Friends

Throughout this season, I always had a friend or family member accompany me during the chemotherapy sessions. I thank them all for taking time out of their busy family lives and for sharing in this part of my survival. During this chapter of my life there was never a day that went by, where I did not receive uplifting and supportive messages, prayers, poems via telephone calls, text and WhatsApp messages, email, letters, cards, and flowers. Sometimes when I was up for visits, I would be taken out or had lunch delivered. I cherished those moments and am forever grateful…

Doing My Research

Researching and educating myself on the type of breast cancer diagnosis I suffered, helped me to come to terms with what I was going through and what I had to do to help myself along with my healthcare team. During my rest days from chemotherapy, I knew that I had to maintain my mind, body, and soul by maintaining a

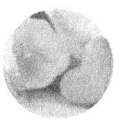

positive outlook, mindset, and a sense of Hope. A positive outlook helped me to better cope with the challenges of chemotherapy.

I found that when I was attuned to my mind, body, and soul, I became more aware of how the treatment was affecting me and this self-awareness led to having better communication with my healthcare team which then enabled them to address my concerns and tailor my treatment as needed. In my opinion When you are attuned to your mind, body, and soul, you are more in touch with your overall well-being and can make decisions and take actions that support your holistic health. Being present in the moment, understanding your emotions, and recognizing when you need to take care of yourself in various ways—whether that's seeking emotional support, practicing self-compassion, addressing physical health needs, or nurturing your spirit through meaningful activities or connections.

Important Tip: *Each individual's journey through a cancer diagnosis is unique and if you do decide to do your own research its crucial to approach information gathering with a critical mindset. Ensure that you're getting information from reputable sources such as medical journals, academic institutions, and well-established cancer organizations. Always discuss any new findings or concerns*

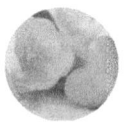

with your healthcare team to get a professional perspective that is tailored to your specific situation.

I was fortunate to always have someone around me, whether it was face-to-face, email, telephone and so on, to talk and laugh with. Although there were many days, I wanted to be shut away and my family and friends understood. I became more aware of my treatments, skin changes, why my finger and toenails became darker, itching skin, why I couldn't use any perfumed soaps, body creams, oils and no perfume or deodorant. The only skincare products I found to help relieve the itchiness I experienced and nourished my body and de-stress my mind was from the Elemis Sp@Home Body Soothing range and in particular, *The Luxury Skin Nourishing Milk Bath*, was a lifesaver. This Luxury Milk Bath has a unique formula that captures the essence of Cleopatra's ancient bathing ritual. Its milk protein base is rich in nourishing vitamins, amino acids, and minerals. Elemis Skin Nourishing Milk Bath contains natural plant collagen, from Oat Extract and Japanese Camellia Oil to feed the skin while keeping skin soft and supple. Skin Nourishing Milk Bath is excellent for irritated, sensitive and excessively dry skin conditions. I still use this product today.

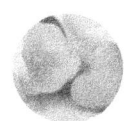

In the third week, I completed my first lot of chemotherapy treatment and started my next session. The second round of chemotherapy, I started to feed my body good nutritional food, took up yoga and stretching exercises as and when I was able to. My spiritual growth grew, and I became so grateful for life, the love and care I had around me. It was now April 2014 and after the third round of chemotherapy, Dr. Quigley informed me I responded well to the chemotherapy treatments and because of that, they were preparing me to have surgery to remove the lump, scheduled for 30th June 2014. It was unbelievable how time was moving, and I was getting prepared to start the next season. My focus was getting through my last few rounds of chemotherapy, healing and keeping strong in both mind and body.

Chapter 3 - Treatment

I was unaware that my body had been invaded and I was unprepared for this season in my life.

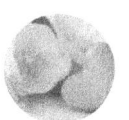

Over the next twelve months from 7th January 2014, it changed from attending social events to numerous hospital appointments. In the blink of an eye, I was faced with a life-threatening disease and nothing was ever going to be the same again. Even with the love and support of my wonderful family and friends, I felt lonely.

Before the next treatment began, there was a further conversation with my Oncologist Dr. Quigley, who explained the various chemotherapy treatments that could take between 7–10 days to have an effect on my body. She went through the various side effects and the 3-weekly assessment. She stressed I must contact the hospital immediately if I developed any signs of an infection. And to help my mental and emotional health I was referred to a psychotherapist and complementary therapist.

To prepare my body, I went through various checks, tests, and scans, all within a one-week appointment. It was an emotional and anxious week. I underwent bone scans, Computer Tomography scans known as CTs, X-rays and various blood tests. The blood tests checked how well my organs like liver and kidneys were working and helped to prevent any complications. The scans were to explore the structure of my heart and examine the size of the tumour. I even had my height and weight measured to help correct any treatment dosage.

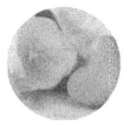

The liver and kidney tests were extremely important, prior to starting chemotherapy, because these organs are responsible for removing the chemotherapy drug from your body, after they have done their job. Blood tests were a normal part of the entire chemotherapy.

Neoadjuvant Chemotherapy

My first course of treatments began with a *neoadjuvant chemotherapy* that was to reduce the size of the tumour. It would then be followed by surgery to remove it from my body. After which I would undergo radiotherapy, a treatment to also kill cancer cells by using high doses of radiation. There were then four courses of Adriamycin Chemotherapy.

Adriamycin Chemotherapy

The Adriamycin Chemotherapy cancer drug was offered as the best treatment option for me because I was diagnosed with primary breast cancer that had spread to my lymph nodes. I was treated with this type of drug to slow or stop the growth of the cancer cells, reducing the risk of breast cancer returning or spreading beyond the breast or lymph nodes under my arm. During treatments, I often felt dizzy, had hot flushes and itchy hands with the added suffering of side effects such as nausea, nose bleeds, cancer fatigue, bone ache and loss of appetite.

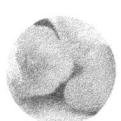

At times, I felt helpless since I was dependent on my family and friends. I was sad, teary-eyed and anxious. I even questioned whether it would all end – „*how much longer would I continue to feel like this?*" And for every three-week session at the hospital, I was truly fortunate to have a family member or friends attend every visit with me. Although I felt lonely, I was grateful that there was never an occasion when I was alone.

Docetaxel

There were four courses of *Docetaxel,* a treatment used to treat breast cancer. This treatment was also administered via a drip in my arm. This treatment was nasty! I had terrible side effects, experiencing excruciating stomach pains, and my white blood cells being extremely low. I even contracted an infection. As a result, I remained in hospital for one week while waiting for my white blood cells to increase. This shook me. I was an emotional wreck, uncertain of how to process what I was going through, but this was when I found strength and said enough was enough. I would not be giving up, and this cancer diagnosis would not defeat me. So, I began to re-educate myself by researching about white blood cells and what I needed to do to prevent them from being low again. White

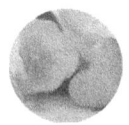

blood cells are the cells of the immune system and protect the body against both infectious diseases and foreign invaders.

On my second round of Docetaxel chemotherapy, it left me in complete agony and I remember lying in bed with stomach cramps which felt like contractions. I keeled over at home and Mauray rushed me to Queen's Hospital in Romford. I was seen immediately, put on a drip and remained in hospital for one week. I had contracted a bacterial infection – *neutropenic sepsis*- *a* life threatening complication to anti-cancer treatment. I was scared. My body was weak, but I was given intravenous antibiotics and began to feel better.

Herceptin

The Docetaxel treatment was followed by *Herceptin,* and this drug increases the chances of being cured of breast cancer and prevents it from recurring. It was delivered by an injection. At the time, there was a six to twelve-month clinical trial, and I was invited to take part. This trial helped to define whether a shorter period of treatment time was effective and what the side effects were.

My white blood cells were low, due to the medical treatments. However, my dietary changes helped to strengthen my immune system, allowing me to feel comfortable. By the time the Herceptin

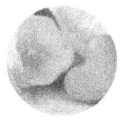

trial began, I was comfortable taking part. The trial allowed me to play an active role in my own health care, as well as, give something back to the medical specialists; more importantly, to help future and potential patients, because of the additional treatments and my hospital check-ups during the trial, I was closely monitored and my hospital care was extended to 10 years instead of the usual five.

During my chemotherapy sessions, I met some lovely people. One such person was Jodie Fitzgerald, and we eventually became great friends. Sadly, she had a second bout of breast cancer and left this earth in November 2016. I was devastated. We used to meet at Lakeside Shopping Centre, for coffee and regularly spoke on the phone, chatting and laughing. She was a beautiful soul and I do miss her. She was such a positive, bubbly and inspirational person and adored her daughters and grandchildren. She loved life, always laughing. I love life and laughter, and I guess this was why we immediately connected, and the two years of our friendship felt like a lifetime. Continue to rest in eternal paradise, Jodie Fitzgerald.

During treatment for breast cancer, I suffered the side effects of chemotherapy and radiotherapy. However, I came through with the help of Breast Cancer Now, the research and care charity. I attended workshops and seminars organised by the charity as I needed their

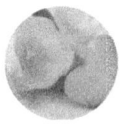

specialist and professional guidance on how to live my life, after a breast cancer diagnosis, including treatment. I needed to know what I could do to protect, not only myself, but my family and friends and if it was not for the support of my breast cancer ambassadors, I may have given up. They made the journey, painless, at times.

I attended workshops and seminars and met other women who were experiencing different types of breast cancer. That was such a breath of fresh air for me. Interacting with others under the same umbrella but with different experiences, helped me to come to terms with my own experiences. During these seminars I met two beautiful souls – Debs Carton and Caroline – and we became great friends, being involved in Breast Cancer campaigns together.

Tip: *It was important to surround myself with women and men who understood the pain, discomfort, and hurt, I was going through. It was then I knew that I was not on my own.*

The Surgery

The following four months were spent experiencing different effects of chemotherapy and responding well to the drugs. The time arrived

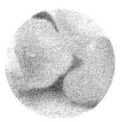

for surgery to remove the cancer tumour. A lumpectomy which was situated in my right breast and the lymph nodes under my arm. The surgery was scheduled for 30th June 2014, four days after my 55th birthday and two days after Leona and Joel's wedding. I was so happy and grateful I was well enough to be part of my family's special occasion. My birthday was lovely and my niece's wedding was stunning.

My surgeon – Mr. Ojo, a Consultant General and Breast Surgeon – explained the procedure. Having learnt from my experiences, I asked questions and conducted my own research on Mr. Ojo and the surgery. I needed to know how long he had been a surgeon and how many breast cancer surgeries he had performed successfully. The answers made me happy and comfortable, and the night before the surgery, Mauray dropped me off at the hospital. Although I was anxious, apprehensive and scared, he ensured I was comfortable. The next day was the morning of the surgery, Mr. Ojo paid me a visit. He was kind and said I would be his second patient and that a member of his team would come to collect me around 11am. He went through the procedure again, reassuring me that everything would be fine, and I was not to worry. Although I still felt anxious and scared, I had faith and trusted Mr. Ojo. I also knew I needed to overcome

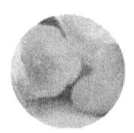

those feelings because I had to get rid of the tumour. I calmed myself, seeking peace with prayer and reciting uplifting affirmations from my little prayer and recovery book.

Eventually, an anaesthetist nurse came and wheeled me into the operating area. He was quite pleasant, asking me a few questions like my name and date of birth. He was shocked when I told him I had just turned fifty-five and wanted to know the secret of looking youthful. He was so surprised that he gathered a few other team members to say how young I looked! Afterwards, he injected my vein on the back of my hand which contained the liquid to send me to sleep. I started to feel light-headed and the next thing I knew I was laying in the recovery room. Mr. Ojo came to visit along with a specialist nurse, and he explained that the operation went well. I started crying, and this time on the nurse's sleeve. She was probably saying: *"Pull yourself together woman"*. But I was just happy and filled with gratitude and thanks.

I guess I must have felt exhausted and relieved that the operation had gone well, and the tumour and lymph nodes had been removed. I stayed overnight and was discharged the following day. Before being discharged I was given pain relief medication, and given a breast care patient leaflet which discussed what you can expect after

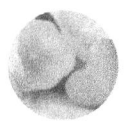

breast cancer surgery and which gave some general information and advice about the following:

Recovery Time

Many people are surprised at the length of time it takes to get over an operation. Most people feel tired, vulnerable and insecure when they first go home. You can also feel frustrated by not being able to do all the things you want to do. Try not to set yourself big tasks. Remember to rest – it is a big part of your recovery. Resting on the bed is more relaxing than in a chair. Try to "pace" yourself and take things „one step at a time". There may be times when you feel isolated or are struggling to come to terms with your emotions. This is a common feeling and there is no right or wrong way to feel. Everyone is individual and will experience different emotions at different times during their recovery. Try to let your family and friends know how you are feeling so they are able to support you. It can also help to discuss it with your breast care nurse or specialist. Psychological / counselling services are available but in high demand with a long wait. Your breast care nurse can refer you to Talking Therapies if appropriate. The "someone like me" telephone support service via breast cancer now offers a service with a volunteer who has "been there too".

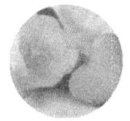

The Healing Process

After your operation, you may have a clear waterproof adhesive dressing on your breast wound or steri-strips (paper skin closures) and a white soft dressing on your armpit wound. The white dressing can be removed when you go home. The clear waterproof dressing and the steri-strips should stay in place and are usually removed in the clinic at your follow-up appointment. You can shower and pat the area dry gently but avoid a bath. Use an unperfumed soap and avoid deodorant until the wound is completely healed. The stitches used are dissolvable, but occasionally, the stitch ends may need to be trimmed. It is quite normal to feel some discomfort, tingling or numbness around the wound. Sharp or shooting pains are often noticeable 7-14 days after surgery. You may notice that the area around the scar is hard and lumpy; this is part of the healing process and will go. If you feel sore or uncomfortable, you may take painkillers following the recommended dosage. If you experience severe pain, contact your GP or ask the advice of the breast care nurses.

Haematoma

After a few days, you may have more stiffness and discomfort as you begin to move your arms more. You may notice a swelling around

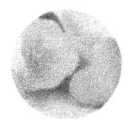

your wounds. This could be due to a collection of blood but doesn't mean you are bleeding. This may not be a problem and there is no cause for concern. If you are uncomfortable or concerned, please contact the breast care nurse for advice.

Infection

In some cases, a wound may become infected. If your wounds become red with increased swelling or discharge, see your GP as you may need antibiotics.

Bras

We suggest that you wear a supportive bra when your drainage tubes have been removed. You can do this in the hospital or wait until you get home. Wearing a bra will help support the wound and will make you feel more comfortable. An old bra may be more comfortable at this stage. Under-wired bras may irritate so are best avoided, though it is possible with some types to slip the wire out of the affected side to make it more comfortable. Sports bras are particularly good, as long as they are not too tight or constricting.

Fuller breasted women may wish to wear a soft bra at night for the first few weeks. If you feel that the area is too sensitive to wear a

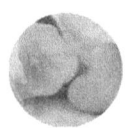

bra, then a cropped top or maternity sleep bra may provide a little support until you are able to manage a bra again.

Lymph Node Surgery

Introduction

The aim of this surgery is to find out whether the cancer has spread beyond the breast. This is done by removing one or more lymph nodes from under your arm on the same side as the affected breast. Lymph node biopsy and dissection has two main purposes. It removes the breast cancer that may have spread into the armpit (axilla). And it allows the surgeon to stage your cancer by learning how far the cancer has spread.

After Surgery

There are a number of sensations you may experience following lymph node surgery. Numbness and soreness under the arm are very common. Your upper arm may become sensitive to the touch. These sensations are due to unavoidable damage to small nerves in the arm during the operation. They will recover and repair, but this does take a number of weeks or even months. Occasionally, pain and unpleasant sensations can persist under the arm despite simple treatments. If this is the case then you should contact your GP,

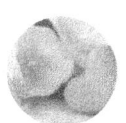

breast care nurse, or mention it at your breast cancer follow-up appointment. If it is particularly troublesome and does not respond to treatment, then a referral to a pain specialist and/or physiotherapist may be required. The arm is often more uncomfortable in the evenings when you are tired. Supporting your arm on a pillow often helps and remember to take painkillers if you need to. Wait until your wound has fully healed before using deodorant; roll on deodorant is better than a spray.

Seroma

A seroma is a build-up of fluid in or around your armpit. You may notice that your armpit or breast becomes swollen or hard and discoloured. If the swelling becomes large enough to cause pain or tightening in the area, it means the fluid needs to be removed. If you experience problems with fluid collecting outside of the seroma clinic hours, you should contact your breast care nurse or the hospital where you had surgery for advice.

Lymphoedema

Keeping your arm in good condition will help to prevent lymphoedema, which is a swelling of the arm on the side where you had your surgery. Lymphoedema is caused by a blockage to the lymph drainage from the arm after the surgery. The blockage could

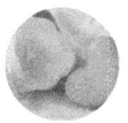

be due to the removal of some of the lymph nodes or scarring after surgery. Lymphoedema may develop at any time after surgery – even years later. Sometimes, the arm does not develop lymphoedema, but the breast or chest wall can be affected by this problem. Similar symptoms of swelling and puffiness of the wound can occur together with feelings of tightness. Again, if you have any concerns, contact your breast care nurse.

Tips for looking after your skin

- *It is important to look after the texture of your skin by keeping it well moisturised. Dryness can cause cracks in the skin, which are ideal places for germs to get in.*

- *Treat small cuts and grazes promptly by cleaning well and applying an antiseptic cream. If the area becomes red, hot, swollen or inflamed, you should consult your GP as you may need antibiotics.*

- *Try and prevent insect bites by using an insect repellent.*

- *Wear gloves for washing up or gardening to try and avoid injury to the hand on your affected arm.*

- *Take care when cutting your fingernails. Wear a thimble for sewing.*

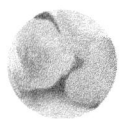

- *Protect your skin from sunburn.*
- *If you feel that your arm is becoming puffy or swollen, contact your breast care nurse.*

I was so grateful for the hospital's support before, during and after.

I had Lymph node surgery. My physiotherapist showed me exercises to do to help improve my movement and prevent arm and shoulder stiffness and I was given an exercise leaflet with the necessary exercises to follow. These exercises included a daily routine of arm lifts and elbow pushes to prevent lymphoedema.

Mauray collected me from the hospital that afternoon and I cannot recall how I was feeling apart from being lethargic. However, I do know that I was looking forward to stepping out of the hospital doors and into my own surroundings, where I would feel more relaxed and comfortable. Obviously, I felt pain and discomfort due to the lymph nodes being removed and numbness around the breast area. I was thankful that I kept my breast and was relieved that part of this season was over. I had to keep a positive mindset to be well enough for the next part of the season – radiotherapy treatment. I kept my mind active by researching how to prepare for radiotherapy, and it helped. I have always believed it was important to educate oneself on any procedure one was about to experience.

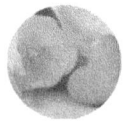

Denial to Acceptance

To gain an understanding of what may or may not happen to one's body.

Three weeks after my operation, I began three weeks of daily radiotherapy treatment, followed by physiotherapy. The effects of radiotherapy were a painful and awful experience, I suffered sore, peeling dry skin, and there were days that I could not lift my arm. The pain was so excruciating and there were days when I was in constant, silent tears. On contacting the hospital, they explained that what I was experiencing were part of the side effects and it will slowly ease. They prescribed a petroleum cream for me to use for my dry and sore skin however, I decided to use the Elemis Skin Nourishing Milk Protein Base collection creams and this helped to relieve the soreness and dryness. Eventually my skin quickly healed and I felt relieved from the effects of the radiotherapy treatments. When I was in my early thirties, I remember suffering with eczema in the creases of my arm. My GP prescribed a steroid cream that irritated my skin after one use. I stopped using it and, coincidentally, around this time I came across QVC Shopping Channel advertising a nourishing moisturising cream that relieves itchiness, eczema etc. It was advertised as being safe to use on babies and I thought if it was safe for babies, it was definitely going to be safe for me. I immediately

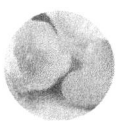

made a purchase. Once I started using this miracle cream, my eczema cleared up within days. I became a big fan of *Elemis* products.

With the invasive treatments over, I am now on *Letrozole*. A tablet that can help control how the cells and organs work, reducing the hormone - oestrogen – and helps prevent the cancer returning. I needed to take this daily until 2024. I was also prescribed *Risedronate Sodium* that I took once a week, this helped my bones stay as strong as possible and calcium tablets for healthy bones. In addition to taking my prescribed medication, I took multivitamins, collagen drink, walk, dance and regularly do yoga and strength *resistance exercises.*

Eventually, Dr Quigley, my Oncologist summoned me to attend psychotherapy sessions.

I had misconceptions about psychotherapy sessions. At first through ignorance, I felt hesitant and reluctant and refused to attend because I thought it was only for "serious" mental health conditions or that it will be a never-ending process. I believed that I felt strong enough to handle and cope with my emotions without the support of psychotherapy. I felt embarrassed and vulnerable about opening about my personal feelings, thoughts, and experiences because I was not accustomed to sharing my emotions with others.

However, I now know that Psychotherapy was part of my cancer treatment plan, and it was natural to feel hesitant or reluctant about undergoing psychotherapy. I am happy and grateful that Dr Quigley insisted on this therapy for me because it supported me emotionally gave me a confidence booster and helped in my recovery to overcome my mental and emotional issues.

Tips on why Psychotherapy is recommended:

Emotional Support: A cancer diagnosis can bring about a range of emotional challenges, including fear, anxiety, depression, and stress.

Psychotherapy can provide a safe space to express and process these emotions, offering emotional support during a difficult time.

Coping Strategies: Psychotherapy can equip you with coping strategies to navigate the emotional and psychological impact of cancer and its treatments. Learning healthy ways to cope with stress and anxiety can enhance your overall well-being and resilience.

Quality of Life: Addressing emotional and psychological distress through psychotherapy can improve your quality of life. By

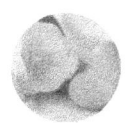

addressing issues related to anxiety, depression, and other emotional struggles, you may experience an enhanced sense of well-being and life satisfaction.

When I was first diagnosed with cancer, I was in doubt and denial. I had trouble believing or accepting the fact I had cancer. I was overwhelmed during this chapter of my life because I had lost control. My normal routine was disrupted by doctor visits and appointments, and I needed to turn down social events because I was either too ill, tired, or exhausted, and felt uncomfortable with my body image. I really felt guilty and wondered if I was going to live.

This season of my life was a life-changing experience, but despite the stress, depression, fear, anxiety, and loneliness, I had a sense of hope. It enabled me to be a kinder person to myself and live a better life than I have ever done before. I found having gone through cancer made me want to live. I made new choices, appreciated and respected life more, and I have come to value and realise how precious it was to embrace my life every day. You want to explore and live life with an attitude of gratitude. I am not just surviving, I am thriving and most importantly, I will do anything in my power, to raise the awareness of breast cancer and to help others.

Denial to Acceptance

Yvonne, my cousin, was incredibly supportive from the first day I was diagnosed, and she would phone every day to check up on me. I remember when chatting with her, I had said that I would not take the chemotherapy. She just listened, never judging me. However, after conducting my own research about chemotherapy and having discussions with other women who had experienced breast cancer and my breast cancer nurse, I decided if I wanted to live, chemotherapy was my best option. Especially, since the cancer had spread. So, when I relayed that to my cousin, she was very relieved.

Mauray was extremely helpful, supportive, kind, and caring, and was my rock during this time. I remember him telling me not to worry, we would fight this together. I was grateful for the support from Mauray's family, my brother Clarence, Sandra, my sister-in-law, nieces, family, friends, relatives, cousins, and co-workers. I sincerely appreciate everyone who sent me kind messages, gifts, flowers, and telephone calls.

Chapter 4 - Recovery

There was never a question in my mind that I was not going to recover from this disease. I was determined to be well again! "I would never, in any way, want cancer again, but it has changed my life for the better"

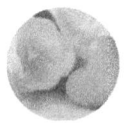

Denial to Acceptance

I became a changed woman, adopting a healthier lifestyle in mind, body, and soul, feeling much better than I have in decades. My skin now glowed, I took regular exercise, strength resistance training, walking, stretching, mediating, laughing, and smiling; reinforcing my body that was once wiped out by chemotherapy. I also learned that having a debilitating disease, like breast cancer, could move and change the goalposts in your relationships. My romantic and personal relationships with a significant other, family, and friends were different, but then I was also a changed woman, not taking anyone or anything for granted. Importantly, I now know that life is invaluable, and living and embracing the moments should be the main thing. I was given a second chance to understand the meaning of life and living life my way.

For that, I am grateful. I cannot go back to the old me but embrace life after breast cancer.

Having breast cancer rocked me, and I expected to return to some sort of normality – what I thought was normal, before my diagnosis. My treatments were all done; thus, I should have been fine, and it was not like that. I had different feelings of anxiety, and the fear of the cancer recurring. Many people think that someone, who is recovering after treatment finishes, is fine. But in their head, they are

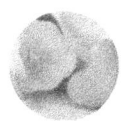

still going through it. January 7th was the date of my diagnosis, and an eternal reminder of what I had been through.

So, in realising how fortunate I was in recovering, I still needed to find a way to cope with my emotions. I took the opportunity to interact with other women, and they were comforting, caring, and compassionate. They were understanding and really helped me along my journey. I attended information sessions and workshops and went on pampering days. In those pampering sessions I learnt how to wear eyeliner and eye shadow and apart from lipstick and mascara, I was never really into make-up, before my diagnosis. As I was not that brilliant at applying, since breast cancer affected my quality of life – emotionally, mentally, and physically – I knew I somehow needed to boost my self-confidence but could not do this alone.

Breast Cancer Care Models

In 2015, I applied to be a model ambassador for Breast Cancer Care now known as, Breast Cancer Now. This event was about celebrating courageous women, stepping out in style onto the catwalk, following a breast cancer diagnosis.

I was turned down and heartbroken, and I now know, it was not my right time. In 2016, I applied again for the show, and this time I was

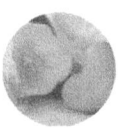

chosen. At the event, I met thirty lovely women and two men who were either breast cancer survivors, going through treatment or had just recently finished treatment. To this day, I'm still friends with them. We share a WhatsApp group, where we share concerns, laughter and organise champagne lunches. On reflection, if I was not diagnosed with breast cancer, I would never have met these wonderful caring, courageous, supportive and fun-loving people.

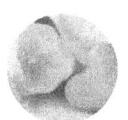

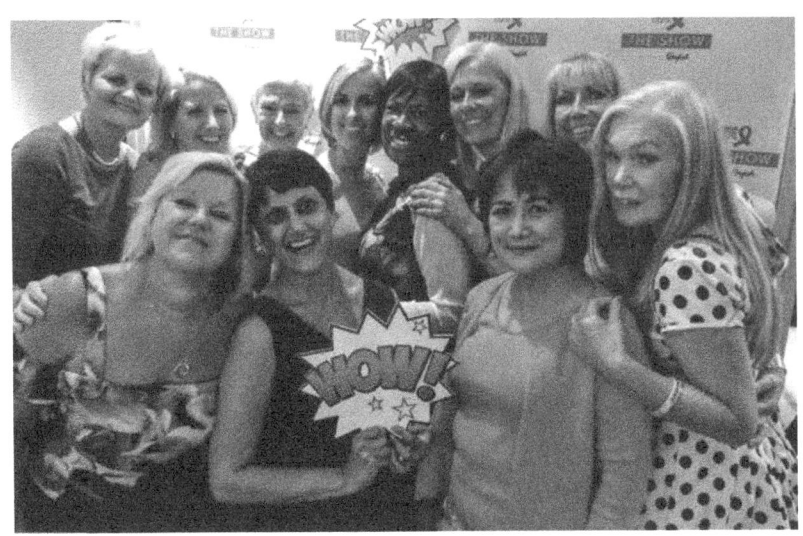

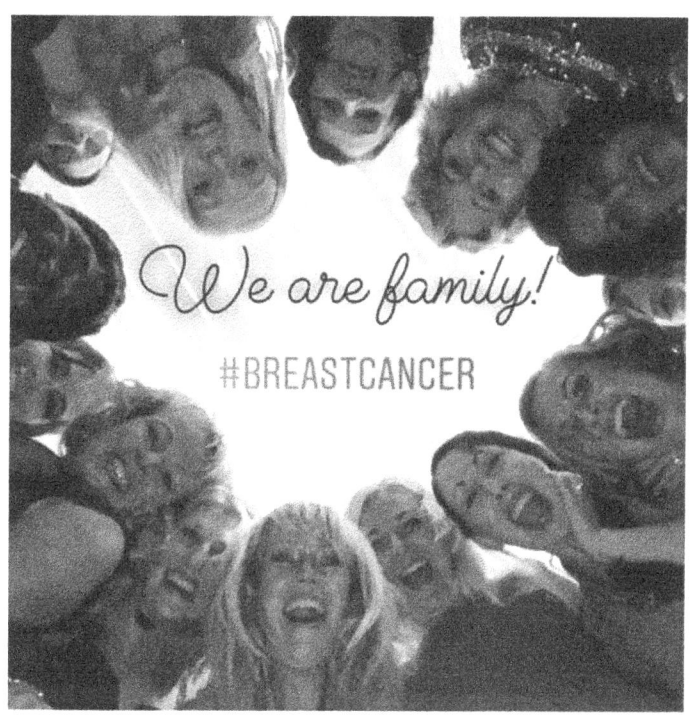
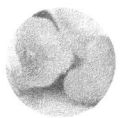

Cynthia Langdon

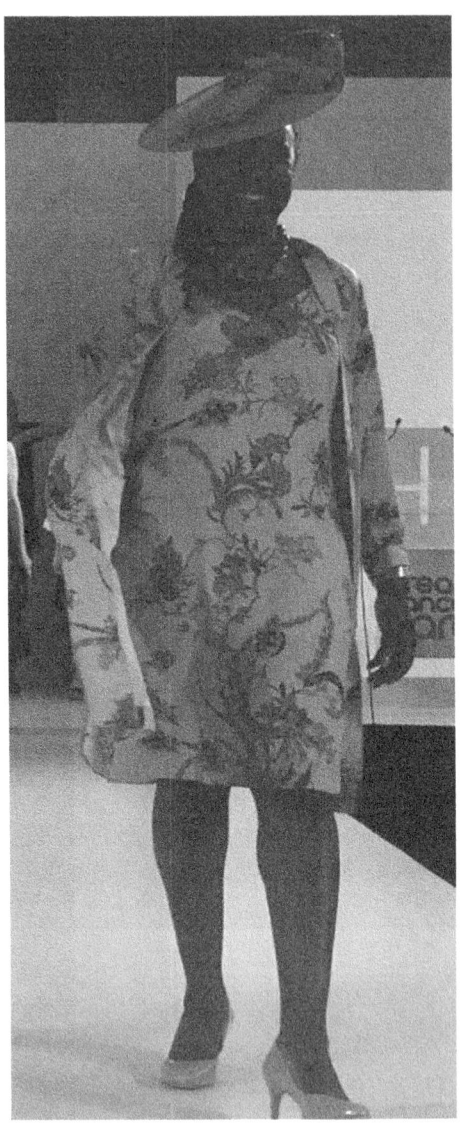

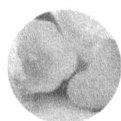

Breast Cancer Care (now known as Breast Cancer Now)

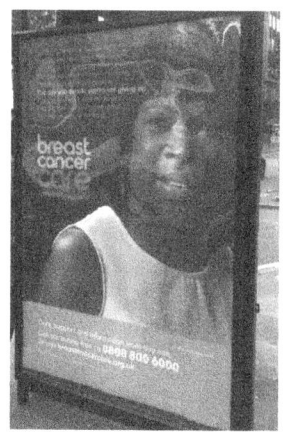

In September 2016, I became one of Breast Cancer Now's Campaign ladies, raising breast cancer awareness, predominantly for women of colour. All over London and Scotland, my face was on billboards and tube stations advertising; in Scotland, I was even on the back of buses! Something good had come out of the breast cancer diagnosis, and I was now helping to raise breast cancer awareness. It is devastating to know the number of women and men who are affected by this disease.

When faced with a breast cancer diagnosis and when experiencing the dreadful treatments, one can feel low, depressed, lose interest in their physical appearance withdraw from others, be tearful, irritable, moody or suicidal. There are charities that offer so much support and hospitals who tender complementary therapies, such as aromatherapy, massage and reflexology, talking therapies, counselling and psychological support; everything excellent for our mind, body and soul.

I turned to Breast Cancer Now, (formerly known as Breast Cancer Care), a research and care charity. This wonderful organisation

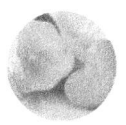

provided information and support, helping me to recover and become the confident, strong, and the inspiring woman I am today. Profoundly, grateful to this organisation, I learnt that nobody needed to go through breast cancer or the treatment alone and it really helped me to interact and share feelings, emotions, and concerns with others. I highly recommend that if you or anyone else you know is dealing with this disease do so with the support and guidance of this or any other such organisation. This would assist immensely. I realised that one word from someone who cared, could boost my confidence and this came through Breast Cancer Now. I found that expressing my concerns or recording my thoughts in a journal helped to ease my worries. They taught me to keep busy, do activities or simply get out of the house, all of which helped me to stay busy. In the end I decided to help myself and others, by volunteering with Breast Cancer Now (www.breastcancernow.org).

Owning My Recovery

Approximately, one year after my diagnosis, I was referred to the Clinical Genetics Unit at Great Ormond Street. Since I had suffered breast cancer at the age of 53 and my mum had bilateral breast cancer in her late 50s early 60s as a precaution, I was tested to ensure that there were no strong genetic links putting me at risk of

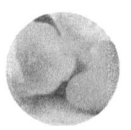

inheriting the BRCA1 and BRCA2 genes[2]. Fortunately, there were no signs of me inheriting these genes.

As I continued on this season, I wanted to own my recovery. My hair grew back, soft and curly and I stopped wearing head wraps and bandanas. I changed to wearing different wigs: short bobs, long flowing, long plaits, cornrows, black, brown, or red. You name it; Cynthia was rocking her new styles. Wigs were something I never dreamt of wearing, before the diagnosis. However, I became very versatile with them and my hair, and loved it. I discovered that wearing wigs made me look and feel more like myself. They made me more confident, and I felt more in control of how I looked. Wigs do require a bit of extra care to prolong life, and they can become expensive, especially, if you get them made to fit you. After a few years, as my hair started to grow back, I decided to go for the low maintenance look and keep my hair neatly cut short.

---

[2] *The name "BRCA" is an abbreviation for "Breast Cancer gene." BRCA1 and BRCA2 are two different genes that have been found to impact a person's chances of developing breast cancer. Every human has both the BRCA1 and BRCA2 genes. Further explanation can be found on the Breast Cancer Now website: „Bilateral breast cancer – Cancer that occurs in both organs"*

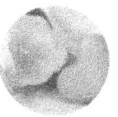

Cynthia Langdon

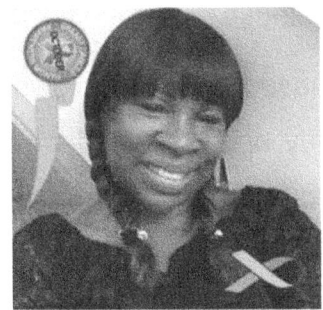

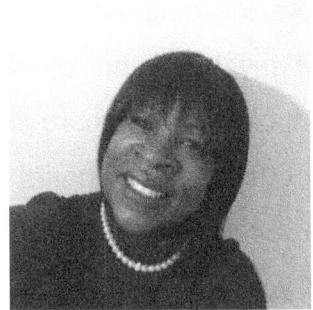

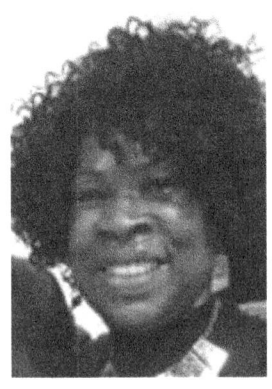

Denial to Acceptance

Sadly, my hair never grew back to its previous life, before the cancer, but who cares! My heart is beating, I am grateful to be alive and sharing my story to the world. Having a lack of hair was something that the "old Cynthia" would have stressed about. My nails and toenails had also changed to a dark colour, and I began to see that return, and so no longer needed to wear any nail varnish to disguise them. It was only after my treatment had stopped, and I started to heal, that I realised the massive changes my body had gone through. During these times, and with the changes in my body, I never believed I would get over the trauma, but I did.

I felt drained after my treatment, and at times, my ability to communicate with others (like, with my loved ones) had weakened, even though they were overwhelmingly supportive. They probably felt I was being ungrateful, and I also wondered whether I would be physically fit again, as well as fearing the cancer returning. I now know that I experienced chemotherapy brain, as I became forgetful, disorganised and constantly crying, to the point where the mention of the word "cancer" would make me cry.

To this day, when I hear the word, I feel emotional, since it takes me back to when I was diagnosed. I now know that this is part of the process of healing. After treatment, it was important to remember, it

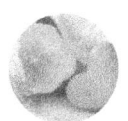

would take time to recover physically and mentally and allow the body and mind to heal.

Breast cancer is very scary. The word *"cancer"* is frightening since we believe that our destiny has ended, yet, leaving this earth is inevitable for us all but at what stage? We have no control over that! If we are faced with this misfortune of getting the disease, we can do our best to fight it, heal and recover to go on, to live a wonderful, beautiful and blessed life. I recovered from breast cancer treatments and because of this, my passion is not just to help you recover from breast cancer but to help raise awareness of breast cancer. Early detection can save lives. I promise to do my utmost best to support, guide and encourage anyone reading this book. R*emember "YOU"* must teach you how to help yourself. Everybody will go through something that has changed them in some way and they may never return to the person they once were. If I could name one thing that breast cancer has taught me, it is to devise a plan for coping with the different emotions. The importance of having an open mind and trying different strategies that work best. Most importantly, I cannot stress this enough…open up to friends, family, a counsellor, therapist, someone you feel comfortable with about any fears or concerns.

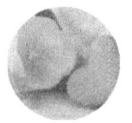

Chapter 5 - Lifestyle Changes Days

I surmounted and braved one of the toughest ordeals I have ever had to face

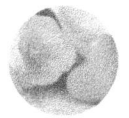

A New Direction

Five months after treatments, it was time to get away and celebrate with a special trip. I desperately needed a holiday because so much of my daily life and mental energy revolved around digesting every fragment of information, treatment, and hospital visits. I decided to plan a short trip to sunny Malta. Planning this trip gave me something to look forward to and took my mind back to pleasant thoughts, daydreaming about warm beaches and relaxing by the pool. Arranging this trip took my mind off worrying about the gloomy and, sometimes, bothersome treatments I had to endure.

Before going, I checked with my hospital team about any precautions I needed to be aware of, and whether I needed to pack anything special. Although I was travelling to a warm, sunny country, I was advised to pack long-sleeved, lightweight tops and pants to prevent exposure to the sun on my skin. I was encouraged to wear light compression socks to help support any pressure associated with air travel and to prevent any swelling.

During breast cancer surgery I also had lymph nodes removed. Therefore, it was important for me, to also wear an arm compression sleeve as a safeguard to prevent the risk of developing Lymphoedema. (*Lymphoedema, a swelling, caused by a build-up of*

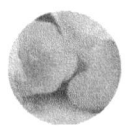

fluid in the body's tissues. Some people develop lymphoedema, after treatment for breast cancer. The swelling commonly affects the arm and can include the hand and fingers. Swelling can also affect the breast, chest, shoulder, or the area on the back behind the armpit. It can occur, as a result of damage to the lymphatic system. For example, because of surgery or radiotherapy to the lymph nodes under the arm and surrounding area. Lymphoedema only impacts the side of the body that was treated. Lymphoedema is a long-term condition, which means that once it has developed, it can be controlled, but is unlikely to go away completely).

(Further information about Lymphoedema can be found on Breast Cancer Now's website)

I received the all clear from my hospital team to travel. Now, my only concern was the cost of travel insurance for my now pre-existing medical condition. A difficult diagnosis should not stop you seeing the world. So, after shopping around for travel insurance I received a reasonable quote that was personalised and tailored according to my needs. Mauray, my partner and I, were on our way to Malta. It was such a wonderful feeling getting away from the cancer diagnosis experience and surroundings and investing quality time to celebrate. No hospital visits, no needles, just pure relaxation.

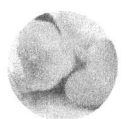

It was important for me to talk about my ex-partner, Mauray. He played a huge part in my breast cancer season. This gentleman cared for me 24/7 and words alone cannot express my sincere thankfulness and gratitude. I was overwhelmed by the care and support given and although Mauray and I were no longer in a romantic relationship, I thank God for putting him in my life. He was my rock and I am truly grateful for our continued friendship.

Friendship is one of the best relationships in the world.

There is a quote, from one of my great idols, Iyanla Vanzant: **People may come into your life for a reason, a season, or a lifetime.** I believe it fair to say that Mauray and I were romantically in each other's lives for a reason and a season.

Iyanla Vanzant, was someone I admired - an American Inspirational Speaker, Spiritual Teacher, Author and Life Coach, and I regularly read daily quotes from her book *"Acts of Faith"*. This not only helped me find peace and energy during this breast cancer season but helped to heal my mind, body, and spirit. I believe it was important to find something that brought comfort, peace and strength, especially when going through a misfortune in health and when experiencing dark days. There were many dark days at times and when Mauray went to work, I used to sit on the edge of the bed and

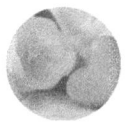

cry uncontrollably. I felt alone…I felt scared…I felt a burden…I was suffering…I was in pain… and I was not in control. Those days, I wished my mum was by my side. She could heal my broken heart. I wanted her arms around me. I wanted her to tell me that all would be well and that what I was growing through would pass. My mum battled with breast cancer, and she would have understood how I was feeling and going through. She would have put that smile back on my face.

A poem for my Mother, Verona

M *is for the Many things she gave me.*

O *is Only that she was growing old.*

T *is for the Tears, she often shed for me.*

H *is for her Heart, as pure as gold.*

E *is for her Eyes that shone so brightly.*

R *is for many Riches; she gave to me.*

I wanted my mum to wipe my tears. I just wanted to feel her love and warmth and her comfort. Then, when I read scriptures from books like: T.D. Jakes, *"Holy Bible, Woman, Thou Art Loosed!"* (given to me as a special gift) provided peace, comfort and strengthened my faith.

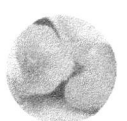

Reading daily inspirational and healing quotes from pocketbooks like: Penelope Sachs, *"Take care of YOURSELF"* and *"Inspiration and Advice for Body and Soul"* and Paul Wilson's *"The Little Book of SLEEP";* helped relieve my pain and anxiety and increased my confidence. They gave me strength, upliftment, energy, comfort and a sense of peace. Reading was so important to me because it gave me hope and was part of my healing process.

Mauray and I arrived in Malta in October 2014. We stayed at the Radisson Blu Resort & Spa Hotel. The hotel was in a beautiful quiet area, relaxing with the sun shining every day – exactly what I needed and wanted. We enjoyed some well-deserved pamper days and there were days when we just strolled and took in the views. But since my energy levels were still low, most of our days were spent chilling, eating, chatting and laughing by the pool. I wore my beautiful, colourful *tankinis* and always made sure I put on my beach cover-up cotton lace long-sleeve dress and sarongs. Our time in Malta was spent reflecting on the past ten months and on a bright future.

Tip: *It is important to reward yourself, at the end of treatment. I thoroughly enjoyed our week in Malta. I went through stressful*

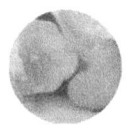

situations and my reward was taking off for some well-deserved pampering. No hospitals, needles or tubes, just pure relaxation.

The day had arrived for us to leave Malta and head back to the UK. Whilst packing I was already feeling the post vacation blues. I was feeling sad due to the changes the cancer diagnosis had caused. I worried about my body image, scars, and fear that the cancer would return, plus about the future. While on holiday, I had the opportunity to distance myself from the hospital visits, needles, and tubes! And for a short while I felt in control of my life again. However, I knew I had to do my best to overcome those doubts and adapt to a new and normal life. When I looked at myself in the mirror, I thanked God for my breasts. I thanked God that the tests confirmed I only needed to have surgery to remove the tumour and there was no need for breast reconstruction. I began to appreciate my body more than ever and was just so grateful to be in the land of the living. When I was told I had a breast cancer diagnosis and would be having chemotherapy for six months followed by surgery, then radiotherapy, it felt like my entire world had come crashing down and the following months of treatment and surgery would never end!

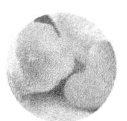

I reflected on the unbelievable support, care, and kindness of everyone - the NHS, my healthcare team, my physiotherapist, my psychotherapist, my therapeutic and wellness therapist, and my personal yoga teacher. The lovely friends I made during this season, my family, friends, relatives, co-workers – Everyone held a special place in my heart because of their individual roles, contributing to my care of healing and recovery. Their support helped me to reduce depression and stress, my improved posture, increased my flexibility, relaxation, and elevated my happiness to overcome problems.

Though many of my friends and family may not have had any understanding of what I was experiencing, they helped to pull me through. I often thought, *"How were they feeling?"* Because they also experienced emotions of distress, anxiety, fear, sadness and frustration. Though the focus tended to be on the person going through treatment, loved ones and carers needed support and comfort too. It was important for them to lean on trusted friends. It was essential that they do not suffer in silence, in relation to their own concerns or fears. Many support groups and online community groups offered support to those struggling with their emotions.

Denial to Acceptance

The past 10 months felt like a dream. It was surreal. I was in doubt and denial and convinced myself I was not ill and that the diagnosis would go away. But when I looked at my body and the trauma it went through, I was grateful to have survived everything. Having the diagnosis taught me how short and precious life was and that in a blink of an eye everything could change, without even realising. My breast cancer diagnosis made me appreciate what I had and how I wanted to live and enjoy my life to the fullest.

Going through my experience, I felt several emotions - low moods, fear, disbelief and distress. However, reading and listening to music played a big part in my healing and recovery. Music improved my mood, decreased my pain, anxiety and distress. Music was my therapy; it made me feel good, calm and relaxed. Fast and slow tempos, great rhythm, smooth jazz, lover's rock, reggae mix, Soca and classical. I enjoyed a mixture of genres. Music has a way to put a smile on your face and wrap a loving hug around your heart.

Prior to my breast cancer diagnosis, I believed that I was a healthy human being. Regularly exercising, eating well and having fun. But now I know I did not feed my body with enough of the daily vital nutrients to keep my cells healthy and bones strong. I was unaware my heart was filled with anxiety, pressure and stress! Though, I am

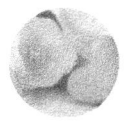

not saying that pressure and stress no longer affect me. On the contrary, I just no longer allow this to take control of who I was and what I chose to do. I no longer tolerate negativity and I certainly do not have negative people around me; I detach myself from negativity. I also became more aware that meditating, journaling, and prayer were the most powerful tools one could use and have in their lives. Now, I meditate and pray daily. It allows me to remain focused, calm, thankful and grateful for what I do have and for whom I genuinely have in my life.

The Important Changes I made

I must say that although my treatments have ended and I am cancer free, it took time to process everything I went through, to recover physically and mentally. What I faced was monumental and took time to come to terms with. It was a bumpy ride and I was OK. My scars have faded, and my life has moved on. I am now living a new normal life. I will never ever be the same as I was before the breast cancer diagnosis, and I am happy and grateful to say that my changes have been a beautiful blessing. I have gained the strength and wisdom of someone, who has faced their worst fears, and my gratitude has become stronger than my anxieties. The breast cancer diagnosis made me realise that I have a purpose! A purpose to co-create and live my happy, joyous and fulfilling life with family, relatives, genuine friends and to genuinely experience it as fully as possible. I have been given that second chance to live life my way and my purpose is to be more present and aware to love deeply, to give immensely, to serve and love others to the best of my abilities. It is to consistently learn, evolve, grow, have tons of fun and become all that I can become.

My Food and Physical Activity

It was important to have a variety of tasty, good food to help with a well-balanced diet that includes protein, carbohydrates, fruit and vegetables. For me, eating essential nutrients was vital since there was the risk of developing osteoporosis or brittle bones because of the chemotherapy treatment and family history. My mum suffered with this and I learnt from reading and educating myself that

Osteoporosis is called a *"silent disease"* because it was not noticeable until a bone broke. As living tissue, to keep them strong, the body broke down the old bone and replaced it with new bone tissue. Therefore, it was essential to train with resistance exercises, especially after undergoing chemotherapy and radiotherapy treatments.

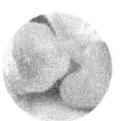

Tip: Exercising does not just mean going to the gym. It means moving your body, walking, dancing (whilst preparing your meals), squatting (whilst cleaning), stretching every day, doing something that you like and enjoy and, most importantly, can smile whilst doing it. During the early days of recovery, apart from walking every day, I also wanted a type of workout that would not leave me exhausted and put stress on my body, especially my arms.

*I found **Imi's Bigan Yoga** (YouTube). There were simple stretching exercises that I could do, sitting on my chair, watching TV. Although these exercises looked pretty simple, they were very effective and made me sweat! I do enjoy going to the gym and attending yoga classes at the gym. It is important to do exercise with a professional teacher/trainer (especially if you are new to exercise and yoga) and others who will continue to encourage and boost your confidence. It is so critical to find and choose an exercise routine that fits into our own individual lifestyle. Moving our body for at least 15 minutes every day is essential for good health, strong bones, healthy cells, stress release and glowing skin. I have learnt to embrace my body for better health and to prevent illness.*

Something I now know I took for granted.

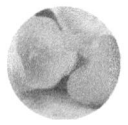

Denial to Acceptance

It was important for me to prevent this disease occurring and I took many healthier lifestyle steps to prevent this by increasing the variety of fruit and vegetables that would help to fight infections and help protect my body from cancers and other inflammatory conditions such as red berries that have powerful antioxidant properties.

To also brighten up my health and support my immune system, I regularly boiled citrus fruit peels, lemon, grapefruit, and orange. They are rich in vitamin C and E and help alkalize one's body. They also contain antioxidants like flavonoids which can protect your cells from free radical damage that puts you at an increased risk of cancer, heart disease, and other illnesses. It is a fact that grapefruit and lemon both regulate blood sugar and help reduce blood pressure. So, introducing them into a daily diet may result in a better-balanced organism. I would usually prepare the citrus peels drink the night before and it would be a great kick start to my day to cleanse my digestive tract and liver.

I began on a variety of dark green leafy vegetables. Rich in minerals, including magnesium, iron and potassium, I love all vegetables. However, prior to my breast cancer diagnosis, I hated the bitter taste of kale but after learning about its benefits, I have come to love this super food and include this in a variety of my delicious dishes at least

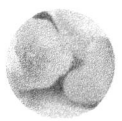

four times a week e.g., stir fries, curries, salads and vegetable pies; the list is endless. Amongst other things kale is shown to be protective against osteoporosis, cancer, and diabetes. High in vitamin A, C, K, Calcium, Iron and it promotes liver health. Kale is known as one of the power foods filled with antioxidants.

I enjoyed eating a variety of fish especially Salmon for Protein/Vitamin D, an excellent source of Omega 3, Fatty Acids that our brain and body needs. Beans and Legumes, heart healthy foods rich in fibre and Vitamins, Protein, Iron, and Potassium. Not forgetting Caribbean dishes that included yam and green bananas. Yams were packed with nutrition, rich in Vitamins, Minerals and Fibre, high in Potassium and Manganese, important for bone health. They also had cancer fighting properties. I grew up with yams and green bananas but ate very little because I did not like them. Now, I reintroduce them into my dishes at least once a week.

I sourced a number of variety of recipes from *The Biblical Nutritionist* (YouTube)

Tip: *There is so much information on healthy food, vegetables etc. It is essential to source what is best for you. Invest in a nutritionist if unsure of what foods can help with lifestyle changes and prevent*

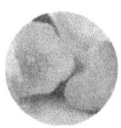

related illness. I find it helpful to seek guidance and support from professionals on how to start a new lifestyle regime. It is also just as important to carry out your own research and decide to make your own choices. - Your Body – Your Better Health

Communicating with Others

After my recovery I decided to join breast cancer support groups, where I would have the opportunity to discuss my diagnosis but I found it helpful to hear about other people's experiences. Although I always received support from friends and family, I wanted to be around people who were going through similar experiences because they had a better understanding of what I was going through. I did not feel so isolated because I found it helpful to connect and share my experiences and concerns without fear of judgement or misunderstanding. These groups provided opportunities to share information, resources, and types of meetings whether in person, telephone or online. Personally, I preferred online and in person. It was normal to feel scared, overwhelmed and isolated after a diagnosis but one can overcome those emotions. Talking to others who knew because they had been there, could make all the difference.

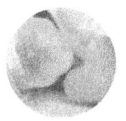

Family

One thing I learnt from this chapter in my life was about healthy and unhealthy communication between friends and family. Communication must be healthy and clear, allowing for small problems to be dealt with easily and the relationship to move on. However, when communication was less healthy, small issues became larger concerns and resentment could grow, fester and result in stress.

Having a life-threatening illness made me realise there were people in my life who secretly hated me and one thing I learned to accept was people came, and people went. Friends you may have made in the past may no longer be around. Family you were expecting to reconnect, were absent. I was disappointed with them, although being estranged; they showed they did not care as much as I thought. It was a sad and painful experience. It was not easy dealing with disappointment from family members because we were wired to believe that family should be there for us no matter what. However, we have flaws and make mistakes. Nobody needs to put up with a relationship that is draining or causing emotional turmoil.

Writing this book has made me realise I was going through challenging situations with close family members. While I failed to

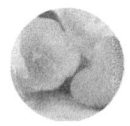

acknowledge the hurt, I was going through over the years, played a part in my illness. I value my self-worth and the support, comfort, and kindness shown from family and friends, who cared and helped me to bounce back. Life could change in a flash, so it was important to be kind.

Having a diagnosis can change your personality in a kind and positive way, so you learn to accept that this can either bring you closer to family and friends or distance you. I have learnt to accept that both are fine. Life can change, that is why it is important to be kind!

And Finally

My breast cancer diagnosis taught me how to live a beautiful life with who and what I have. My life looks different today than I thought it would but it is better than I could ever dream. I am happier than I have ever been and this is because I am living my best life. I am currently single and I do not have children of my own but I am surrounded by lots of love. I am travelling more, running my own businesses, writing my book and have a wonderful circle of family and friends, who love and care that I am happy, and now safe.

I want YOU to be happy too!

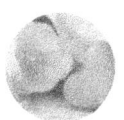

Cynthia Langdon

If you are going through breast cancer, a survivor, carer, or suffering, remember to open-up and talk to someone. You are never, never on your own!

I love my life. It is better than I thought it would be. I am happy, joyful, thankful and grateful to be here.

I am happy to be writing this book with the hope that one person will find some comfort, an answer or information, if faced with a life-threatening illness; because I now know there is sunshine at the end of the dark tunnel.

Chapter 6 - Reflections

Having a cancer diagnosis taught me that the people in your life are the most important, not their looks or what they have. But their warmth, friendship, support, love and many other things they share and give unconditionally

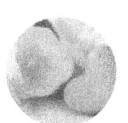

In my previous chapters, I expressed my gratitude to the medical teams that cared for me such as Dr. Mary Quigley, Oncologist. Mr. Ojo, Surgeon, the nursing staff and everyone at Queen's and Bart Hospitals.

In The Workplace

Going through this experience was a rollercoaster ride of emotions, low moods, fear, disbelief, and distress. I found it difficult to cope and my job suffered. As a result, I was unable to continue working for at least 9 months.

When I was diagnosed, I was a full-time employee at a local authority. I remember breaking the news to my team leader over the telephone, from his end there was silence, yet I was laughing since I struggled to accept the devastating news. *"You have breast cancer and it has spread to your lymph nodes, so we have to act quickly".* I was in denial. I was unwilling to believe I was diagnosed with breast cancer. I was hiding away from the fact that this could be true. I was anxious and fearful, so laughing was the only way I could deal with the shock.

The next day on my way into work I met Kash, a colleague and dear friend. When I told him, he stopped in his tracks, and again, I laughed. He said: *"Cynth, this isn't anything to laugh about".* Again,

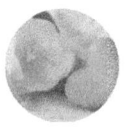

Denial to Acceptance

I knew that, but this was my way of dealing with the news, with the shock, denial, and disbelief. Laughing at my own statement was a release. I did not want to admit I was scared. I was trying to convince myself and everyone around that I was okay. I did not understand what I was about to embark on because I did not want to. I had closed my eyes to cancer.

Telling your boss and colleague you have been diagnosed with breast cancer can bring mixed emotions. You may not know how your boss will react; how supportive the workplace might be. I was not prepared for this conversation, but I knew it was a conversation, only I could do. Fortunately, my colleagues and I had built up a respectful, supportive, working relationship over the years. Therefore, although I knew this news would be devastating, I also knew they would be supportive.

At work, my team leader called me into his office and asked how I was feeling, and how I would like to break the news to the team. I remember him, also saying that they would be devastated, but supportive. I was not sure how I wanted to break the news, but knew it was something I personally had to do. We called them into a meeting room. Some looked puzzled, some asked if I was leaving,

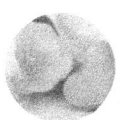

was I pregnant? Had I been promoted? Even, am I getting married at last! Their questions were quite amusing.

We were a close team, who worked well together and supported each other. I plucked up the courage to tell them the reason for the unexpected summons. Their faces expressed sorrow, shock, some bowed their heads; everyone was silent. Smiling, I did my best to lift their spirits by saying, *"I know that I'm going to fight this, I know that I'm not going to allow this illness to control me"*. I did not want to be treated differently; I wanted them to continue making me smile and laugh every day, as they normally did. After I broke the news, I did not remain at work. My team leader insisted, I took the rest of the day to go home and rest. I was fortunate, since throughout this season, my colleagues had been so supportive and kind.

During the times when I was away from the office, they would touch base with me, giving me the latest news or office tittle-tattle (I could always rely on them to give me a good old belly laugh, which eased my pain and sadness at times). There was always some story and whenever I was able to attend work, though feeling poorly would insist on treating me to lunch. I had no appetite, but it was just great, being in their company. These were people I had worked with for over 20 years and to this day, we are still in contact with each other.

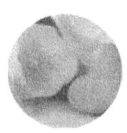

My role, as an Investigation Officer, was intense, interviewing benefit claimants, attending court. However, I enjoyed it and felt I needed to continue my work routine, for as long as possible. I did not want, being diagnosed with breast cancer, to change my life, because I wanted to feel more like myself, and it was great to be around my colleagues.

Finances and Breast Cancer

Money concerns, whether permanent or temporary. It can be particularly stressful, at a time, when you feel less able to cope. Many people with breast cancer do not claim assistance from the Government, because they're unaware of what they're entitled to, and are too embarrassed to ask for help, or find the system complicated. It may not be your first worry, but cancer can be tough on your finances, you may earn less, if you need to stop working or reduce your hours. You may spend more on everyday costs, like heating and travelling to regular hospital appointments. (Unfortunately, because I was employed full time, I was not entitled to any assistance from the government at that time but received free prescriptions and supportive information from *reading the Macmillan Cancer Support Planning & Managing your Finances Booklet).*

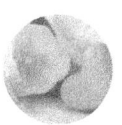

I was worried that my finances would be affected, if I was unable to continue working. How would I be able to pay my mortgage or bills? I tried blocking out this negativity, but this worry still played a big part in my diagnosis. Eventually, I became extremely sick with severe tiredness and aches, experiencing dull throbbing pains in my bones, caused by the adverse effects of the chemotherapy treatments. This affected my performance at work, and I was soon signed off, for over nine months, by my Oncologist/GP and the Occupational Health team, at work. There was a reduction in my pay after six months of being off work. Through my ignorance, I was not prepared and aware that this would happen! Therefore, I made an urgent plea, in writing, to my manager to put me back on full pay. I had suffered a misfortune of being diagnosed with breast cancer that altered all areas of my life. I did not feel it appropriate to suffer a pay cut also. Fortunately, my request was granted and agreed by the Local Authority, Human Resource Department, for a further three months, when I was well enough, to phase back into work. I was truly grateful. I relied on my salary for my upkeep, and having my diagnosis, forced me to think about other ways to generate income.

My colleagues respected my privacy, but would check in on me daily, by using various means, like the telephone or email. I valued their

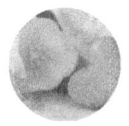

concern and would always express my gratitude, by telling them how thankful I was, for their kindness and support. Even with their own busy lives, they always found that extra time to check in on me, during those dark days.

How My Diagnosis Affected My Family

You may share your news with various family members at different times. This conversation will be tough for everyone, no matter when or where you have it. It can go more smoothly, if you set it up to avoid interruptions or distractions. Although, there is never a perfect moment. Most of us aren't ready to hear shocking news, so we may blurt something out or not say anything at all. Loved ones are not always comfortable hearing shocking news and may have an awkward or unhelpful reaction.

A friend may tell you to cheer up, instead of listening to your fears. A relative may give you advice, share stories, or give their opinion on doctors and hospitals. Not everyone will be comfortable with this news, and this is completely normal. In most cases, people mean well, but do not think about what they are saying…

Sandra

Sandra, my sister-in-law, was the first member of my family, who knew of my diagnosis. I mentioned to her that I had a hospital appointment, (that evening of 7th January 2014), after having a breast examination, a few weeks prior to this appointment. That evening, she popped by, to see how everything went. Her reaction was one of shock and disbelief. An unexpected bombshell, since she was not expecting to hear my devastating news. She was concerned, asking questions about what the consultant said etc. But I cannot remember what my answers were. All I remember is, showing her the multiple leaflets and brochures I was given, by the breast cancer care nurse, to read and digest. I do remember telling

Sandra that I won't be having any chemotherapy treatment. Sandra was very attentive and offered to take me to hospital appointments. She would be the one asking Dr. Quigley questions. When you are told of a breast cancer diagnosis, your mind can become completely blank because you are hearing words nobody wants to hear. I was lucky that Sandra offered to take me to one of my first appointments because whatever Dr. Quigley told me at this time, did not register. Dr. Quigley was so kind and gentle; she really looked after me during this season, both her and her wonderful team.

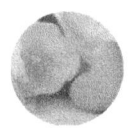

Having Sandra around was comforting. I was scared to tell my brother and asked her to break the news to him. On reflection, this was a bit selfish of me. I was scared to tell my brother Clarence because I was worried about his reaction. However, it was my responsibility to break the news to my brother and not rely on someone else. At the time, I was in disbelief, how could this happen? I knew the conversation would be a difficult one because it would bring back memories of Mum, and I did not want him to be stressed.

Vivienne

Following my visit to the hospital on 7th January 2014, whilst standing outside the hospital grounds reflecting on the consultant's words.

"We have the results of your tests! You have breast cancer, and we need to act quickly because it has spread to your lymph nodes".

That same evening, a bit disorientated, I made a call to Vivienne, one of my school friend's. I struggled to get the words out, about the consultant's diagnosis. Eventually, when I did, she was distraught, since I could hear her tears. In no time, Vivienne was at my home. After which, she would always check in, even going as far as doing research on the Macmillan Cancer Support websites, about breast cancer. She would tell me what she had found, knowing it would help me with my recovery, and always asked if she could post or email

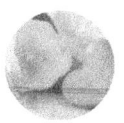

the information she found. Vivienne was a tower of strength, and so loyal, throughout this season. A truly sincere and supportive friend. Vivienne's words were, *"she knew she needed to be with me"* during this season of my life, although there were fears of anxiety, concern, and worry. I now believe my support network hid their true emotions, because I was often upbeat and calm around them, as much as I possibly could be.

Yvonne

Yvonne, my cousin! I broke the news to her, over the telephone. When I told her the news, I felt her expression of shock, as there were a few seconds of silence. Before my visit to the hospital, I did not feel the need to tell my family and friends about the lump, because I was not concerned about it. Yvonne was very attentive during this time, and she was the person I opened up to about my fears of any breast cancer diagnosis. She was concerned that I was in denial and that I had refused to have chemotherapy and radiotherapy treatments. Although, she respected and understood me. Her words of wisdom helped me to come to terms with the news. The realisation of my diagnosis actually sunk in, and I knew I was the only person who could make that decision to accept the treatments needed for me to heal and recover, sooner rather than

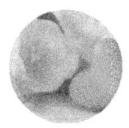

later. Even with her own family commitments, Yvonne offered support and help, she prepared meals, and escorted me to the hospital for my appointments and chemotherapy treatments.

My Brother

This conversation was the most difficult one, because my emotions were all over the place. I was overwhelmed, ignoring my true feelings and was not sure how to proceed. This made it difficult to know how to cope with other people's reactions.

I finally broke the news to my brother, while we shopped at Tesco. For a while, after I told him, he was silent. *How does one tell their family and friends that they have a life-threatening illness?* Especially, as I have always made sure to keep an eye on my health, as far as I was concerned. Anyway, my brother was not one for many words and I knew this news had an impact on him emotionally, because this news was sudden and a shock. I wanted to shield my brother from pain and worry! He had no idea that I had a breast lump, was not aware that I had attended the hospital firstly for an examination much less, receiving results of a breast cancer diagnosis. Emotionally, this news affected him, because it brought back memories of Mum. Nonetheless, on the surface, he handled it well and his love, care, help, and support were unconditional.

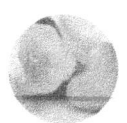

Yvonne Lynch

My friend, Yvonne Lynch, was a former mid-wife. She held my hand from the beginning, offering to attend hospital appointments with me, whenever I needed. Yvonne was devastated, shocked and surprised, but a great tower of strength. She reminded me of how fearful she was, because I had spoken about my Mum's breast cancer to her very often, including how she passed. She was concerned that mine could be hereditary. Her fears were made worse, when I told her that I was not going to have chemotherapy. Instead, I was going down the holistic route. She knew how adamant I was about chemotherapy drugs, but helped with my decision, by encouraging me to research the different alternatives I could take, to heal myself. Yvonne also reminded me of how I had told her about the lump, during our girlie conversations, and that I was in denial, and it could be cancerous. She convinced me to go and get it checked, because she had previously lost a dear friend to breast cancer, a few years before. Through this season of my life, Yvonne said she felt nervous, because of what I was going through.

However, she admired my positivity, calmness, and my thoughts of, *"I can get through this"*, and this made her feel at ease. Yvonne

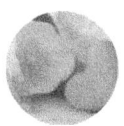

admired how I took things in my stride, and how easy I felt, telling people about this diagnosis, and that I never lost my laughter.

The love from many – names have been withheld due to privacy

It was comforting to know of the many people I could turn to. As I focused on healing, recovering, getting stronger and fitter. My family and friends had a positive impact on my suffering and pain, because during my distress, difficulty, and challenges, they all had hope. They helped me to see that there was sunshine, after the darkness. They kept me going with their comforting words, embracing me, when I needed a hug, showering me with prayers, and filling my heart with smiles and laughter. It was overwhelming, the many friends and family, relatives who sent me well wishes and messages of help, hope, and courage. My cousins from far and wide, the boys from Caribbean International Football Club, the girls from Caribbean International Netball Club. My dearest school friends, from St Angela's Ursuline Convent. My Awesome 2016 Breast Cancer Model Buddies and my best friend Susie (who emigrated from the UK, to Brooklyn over twenty-five years ago). Susie and I have been bosom buddies for over forty years. During my overseas telephone conversations with her I felt her sadness, that she was unable to be close to me, often saying how helpless she felt. What Susie failed to

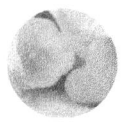

realise was that her telephone calls filled me with encouragement and uplifted me. Whenever I saw her phone number and heard her voice, I would feel elated. Though we were miles apart, she was attentive and unbeknown to me at the time she would make regular telephone calls to my brother, for updates on my progress.

A support network was so extremely important because one cannot get through something so devastating by oneself. I had hope and though there were times when I felt like quitting, my close support network kept me going, with their offerings of help and asking how they could help.

Sometimes, going through a season of suffering and pain, we forget how our loved ones and their families were keeping. Whenever I was in contact with a friend or family member, I always ensured to ask how they and their family were doing. It was not all about me.

Life moves on!

There were times when I found myself, wondering how I was going to make it through. Also, there were times when I felt that I could not go on for another day. However, I also discovered I had courage and strength I never knew I had. I kept my faith and belief that the pain I was going through, was not going to last, unless I allowed it. My friends and family were worried and afraid, some may have even

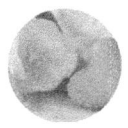

been angry, since all they knew was that I had been a health-conscious person and yet their love, care, support, and laughter contributed to my survival. There was definitely sunshine at the end of darkness.

My Nieces: Leona, Selina, Georgina

Clarence and Sandra, have three grown-up daughters. Although we have a close relationship, I was not sure how to tell my nieces about my diagnosis, so I left this up to their parents. Their initial reaction was of shock and sadness though they were attentive and offered help, emotional support, lent an ear and actively listened to my feelings; that meant a lot to me.

Everyone in my family was devastated, like my eldest niece, Leona, who was planning her wedding, during my illness. This happy celebration took away our sadness because we were looking forward to something grand. My great niece, Saniya. Leona's daughter, who was two years at the time, kept me upbeat. Children are always happy and every time she was around me, she would bring me so much joy, putting a beam of sunshine in my life. Saniya is now nine years old, and I cannot believe where the time has gone! She continues to lift my heart with joy and happiness and keep me on my toes, along with her little brother, my great nephew, Shaylen

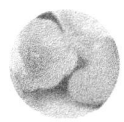

(now five years old). It is important to be around people, who continue to make you laugh every single day and these happy moments also distracted me from the hospital visits, injections, chemotherapy drugs, medication, pain, and sickness.

My faith and determination showed that there is, still life during a cancer diagnosis and with my niece's wedding, a great day of celebration. It helped me so much. I had an aunty role to play, and thoroughly enjoyed her special day. I laughed and had fun with family and friends, dancing the night away. I was so happy and grateful that I was well enough to attend Leona and Joel's wedding, and two days after they got married. I had my last session of chemotherapy, *Monday 30th June 2014.*

I am, and will also be eternally grateful, to everyone in my support network because I also appreciate that they may have felt a mixture of emotions, at hearing the shocking news about me at first, and may have been more worried about me than they let on.

Chapter 7 - A New Life

I love my life because I now do things, I would never have dreamt of doing having had a breast cancer diagnosis

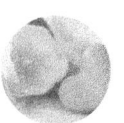

I have been part of several Breast Cancer Now campaigns on the back of buses and billboards, in tube stations and local newspapers. I also featured in numerous issues of the Breast Cancer Now Vita Magazines. I was so honoured to be a part of these campaigns and help to raise breast cancer awareness. I am proud of my big and small achievements since my experience with a breast cancer diagnosis and they fill me with appreciation. I am living my life to the fullest. I have appeared on television soaps, documentaries, films and commercials as a professional supporting artist. I am now an author and met, and still meet, beautiful, uplifting people.

Lessons Learned

They say a worry shared is a worry halved and I appreciate some of us may be uncomfortable in sharing our personal worries. However, there are online forums and message boards where help and support are available. Through my experience it saddened me to know that some people suffer in silence. So, if I can help one person, then I am happy I have done that one thing, supporting someone to face their fears and in doing so, letting them know that they are not alone. *"We can have anything we want, if we're willing to give up the belief that we can't have it,"* said Dr. Robert Anthony.

Denial to Acceptance

I am happy and grateful to know I am responsible for creating my own happiness, by creating how I live my life and who I surround myself with. At times, I found myself fretting about things I may never get to do, if the cancer returned but I began doing them anyway. I now do things to please ME and not feel guilty about saying No! I am so happy and grateful now more than ever, for my life and for my supportive friends and family. The cancer diagnosis changed my body but throughout my experience I have learned to LOVE ME. I am not ashamed of my scars since they simply mean I'm stronger than whatever tried to hurt me and every morning, when I open my eyes and breathe, I give myself a hug and say thank you for this wonderful beginning, to a new day. **Gratefulness** is a powerful word in my life and a word I use every single day.

My experience has shown me that there can be a beautiful, bright, sunshine-filled life at the end of that dark, scary tunnel. It has also taught me that people will leave or enter your new life, and this must not be seen as anything negative since when a job is done, everyone moves on to another season. My quality of life has changed. I survived a breast cancer diagnosis, and this has resulted in a beautiful change in my life. I have made changes to my life and my actions have encouraged my friends and family to live healthier. I

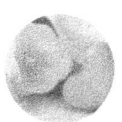

have grown spiritually, feel personal empowerment and have a newfound confidence, to help me achieve my goals. Joining support groups allowed me to gain new friendships and these are connections I may not have made otherwise. I am a strong advocate for breast cancer knowledge and my purpose is to help raise awareness and prevention of this disease. It has been an enlightening journey and I am so grateful for life. It has been a relief and now it is time to Rejoice.

Chapter 8 - Men and Breast Cancer

With permission from Breast Cancer Now. I want to share the importance of becoming knowledgeable about this disease, and it would be amiss if I did not acknowledge that men also develop breast cancer.

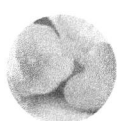

- Although rare, men can get breast cancer. The most common symptom is a lump in the chest area.

- Many people do not know that men can get breast cancer because they do not think of men as having breasts. But men do have a small amount of breast tissue.

- Breast cancer in men is cancer that starts in this small amount of breast tissue.

- Breast cancer in men is very rare. Around 370 men are diagnosed each year in the UK.

- Most men who get breast cancer are over 60, although younger men can be affected.

Signs and Symptoms of Male Breast Cancer

- *A lump in the chest area*

The most common symptom is a lump in the chest area which is often painless.

Other symptoms

Other symptoms of male breast cancer may include:

- Liquid, sometimes called discharge, which comes from the nipple without squeezing and which, may be blood-stained

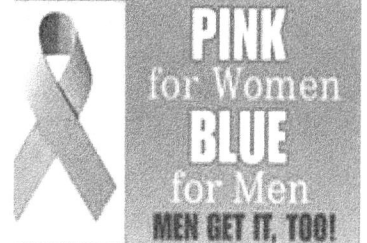

- A tender or inverted (pulled in) nipple

- Ulcers (sores) on the chest or nipple area

- Swelling of the chest area and, occasionally, the lymph nodes under the arm

Causes Of Breast Cancer In Men

The exact causes of breast cancer in men are not fully understood, but certain things increase the risk. The Male Breast Cancer Study is looking at, what might cause breast cancer in men.

What Is The Male Breast Cancer Study?

The Male Breast Cancer Study was established to pinpoint the precise genetic, environmental and lifestyle causes of breast cancer in men. This helps to identify those who are at risk and understand

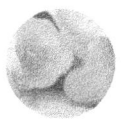

what can be done to lower the chances of developing the disease. The study also aims to identify similarities and differences between breast cancer in men and women.

Other Facts About Causes Of Breast Cancer In Men Include:

Age

Most men who get breast cancer are over 60, although younger men can be affected also.

High oestrogen levels

There is some evidence to show that men are at greater risk if they have higher than normal levels of the hormone oestrogen.

All men have a small amount of oestrogen. High oestrogen levels can occur in men because of:

- Long-term liver damage, particularly cirrhosis
- Obesity (being very overweight)

Radiation

- Men who have had previous radiotherapy to the chest, for example, to treat Hodgkin lymphoma, may have a slightly increased risk of developing breast cancer.

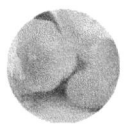

For more support and information on breast cancer in men, call Breast Cancer Now's free Helpline on 0808 800 6000

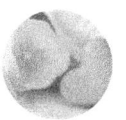

Chapter 9 - Facts and More Information

With permission from Breast Cancer Now, the research and care charity, at the time of writing this chapter, I would like to share some of their recent media facts and statistics, found by their Doctors and Research Managers. (Further information can be found at **https://breastcancernow.org**).

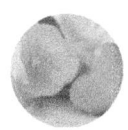

Breast Cancer Facts and Information, 2021

"Around 1,000 women in the UK die each month, from secondary (metastatic) incurable breast cancer and it is vital that people diagnosed with this life-limiting disease can access potential new treatments through clinical trials that could offer them precious extra time with their loved ones or help pave the way for new treatments, for those diagnosed in the future. As such, it is extremely worrying that this survey suggests, the majority of people living with secondary breast cancer in the UK have never been asked by their oncologist about joining a clinical trial. For those, who did enquire about trials, they did not always receive a helpful or positive response. For the thousands of patients, with limited treatment options, clinical trials have the potential to offer much-needed hope for the future. Whilst, the pandemic has disrupted and delayed some trials, as research recovers, we must urgently ensure, everyone with secondary breast cancer has the opportunity to access available clinical trials. We are calling on the NHS across the UK, to commit to and outline a patients' right to be referred to research, underpinned by appropriate support for patients, clinicians, and local systems. Only then, can we guarantee that no patients are left behind.

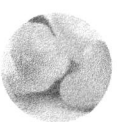

Anyone who is concerned about breast cancer, can get more information by calling Breast Cancer Now's free Helpline on 0808 800 6000 to talk to one of our expert nurses." **Dr. Simon Vincent, Director of Research, Support and Influencing at Breast Cancer Now, 4th November 2021.**

"Around 1,000 women in the UK die each month from incurable secondary (metastatic) breast cancer. We desperately need to learn more about this devastating disease. So that, we can find new ways to improve treatment, care, and support for people living with it. Including those living in fear of a diagnosis. We do not currently know who will develop secondary breast cancer and when. But this new analysis of existing studies, provides helpful insight into who is most at risk. The data shows that people diagnosed with primary breast cancer aged 35 years or younger have the greatest chance of developing secondary breast cancer. The study also highlights the size of the tumour, the type of breast cancer and the length of time since primary diagnosis can impact a person's risk. Secondary breast cancer can develop many years after an initial cancer diagnosis, so it is vital that we understand it better and find new ways to prevent it. The lack of information on people living with secondary breast cancer must

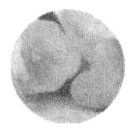

urgently be addressed to ensure each individual's needs are met, so that we can identify the key factors that influence someone's chances of developing the disease. Anyone who is concerned about breast cancer can call Breast Cancer Now's free Helpline on 0808 800 6000 to talk to one of our expert nurses." **Kotryna Temcinaite, Senior Research Communications Manager at Breast Cancer Now, 3rd November 2021.**

"It is encouraging that eating nuts could potentially benefit women who have previously been treated for breast cancer. However, more research is needed into the benefits of nuts, by tracking dietary changes over a longer time, to see if eating nuts can increase breast cancer survival. We know that women, who have completed breast cancer treatment, can find the fear of recurrence, a challenging part of moving forward. Hence, why it is important that we investigate different ways to prevent breast cancer recurrence. This research provides a helpful reminder of the importance of eating a balanced diet, maintaining a healthy weight and being physically active, which can all help reduce the risk of breast cancer recurrence. We would encourage anyone in the UK seeking more information about healthy lifestyle choices, to contact their GP or Breast Cancer Now's free helpline on 0808

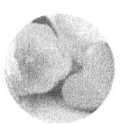

800 6000 for specialist support." **Kotryna Temcinaite, Senior Research Communications Manager, at Breast Cancer Now, 20th October 2021.**

Incidences of Breast Cancer

In the UK, breast cancer incidence rates are lower in women from ethnically diverse backgrounds, including South Asian, Black, Chinese, and mixed groups, when compared to White women. However, women from these backgrounds experience differences in breast screening attendance, the stage and age of diagnosis, survival outcomes, and experiences of care and treatment.

Breast screening

Evidence suggests women from ethnic groups are less likely to attend breast screening, compared to White women in the UK. Lower breast screening uptake may be due to cultural and language barriers and a lack of tailored interventions.

Age at diagnosis

There is a lack of recent data on the age of diagnosis by ethnicity; however, evidence suggests women from ethnically diverse backgrounds in the UK are diagnosed at a younger age than White women.

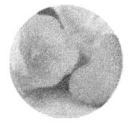

Stage at diagnosis

Black women are more likely to be diagnosed with more advanced breast cancers and breast cancers that have fewer treatment options, such as triple negative breast cancer. Around **25%** of Black African women and **22%** of Black Caribbean women are diagnosed with Stage 3 or Stage 4 breast cancer at diagnosis in England; this compares to **13%** of White women.

Survival

Late-stage diagnosis is associated with poorer survival outcomes in women from ethnically diverse backgrounds, when breast cancer is more difficult to treat. Black women in England, aged 15–64 years, had significantly lower survival from breast cancer at both **one-year (96%) and three-years (85%)** compared to White women **(98% at one-year, 91% at three-years)**. South Asian women aged 15–64 years had significantly reduced survival compared to White women at **three-years (89%).**

Awareness

Studies suggest women with breast cancer from ethnically diverse groups have lower breast cancer awareness and knowledge of symptoms and risk factors, than White women.

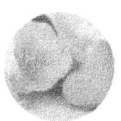

Patient experience

Some evidence suggests that women with breast cancer from South Asian backgrounds report higher levels of depression, anxiety and poorer quality of life measures compared to White women. South Asian and Black women also report a higher level of concern about body image and stronger fatalistic beliefs. The 2019 National Cancer Patient Experience Survey for England highlights that women with breast cancer from Asian, Black, and Mixed Ethnic backgrounds rated their overall care lower than ratings from White women. (For more support and information, call Breast Cancer Now's free Helpline on 0808 800 6000).

What are the Symptoms of Breast Cancer?

Signs and symptoms of breast cancer include:

- A **lump or swelling** in the breast, upper chest, or armpit

- A **change to the skin**, such as puckering or dimpling

- A **change in the colour of the breast** – the breast may look red or inflamed

- A **nipple change**, for example it has become pulled in (inverted)

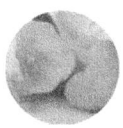

- **Rash or crusting** around the nipple
- **Unusual liquid** (discharge) from either nipple
- **Changes in size** or shape of the breast

On its own, <u>pain in your breasts</u>, is not usually a sign of breast cancer. But look out for pain in your breast or armpit that is there all or almost all the time. One of my symptoms was pain in my armpit which was there almost all the time. I had put this down to muscular strain as I was doing a lot of strength/weight training. I ignored it for an exceptionally long time. Had I been aware this was one of the symptoms of developing breast cancer, I would have acted sooner, rather than later, and maybe, just maybe, the cancer would not have spread to my lymph nodes.

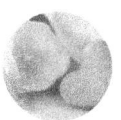

Be Breast Aware

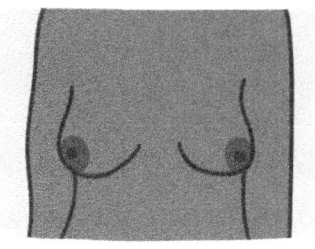 A **lump or swelling** in the breast, upper chest or armpit

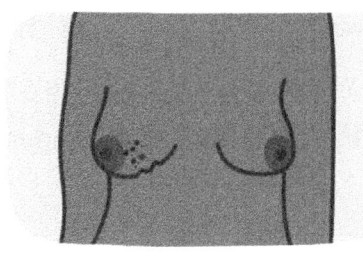 A **change to the skin**, such as puckering or dimpling

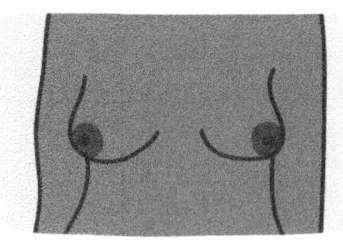 A change in the **colour** of the breast – the breast may look red or inflamed.

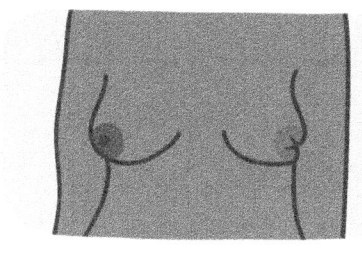 A **nipple change**, for example it has become pulled in (inverted)

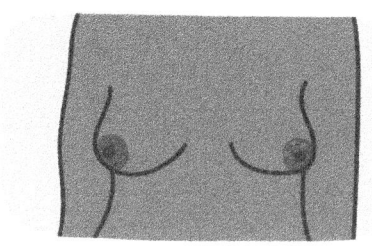 **Rash or crusting** around the nipple

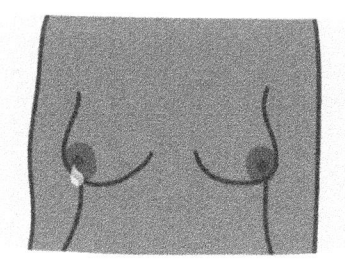 **Unusual liquid** (discharge) from either nipple

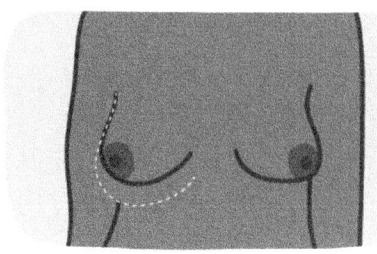

Changes in size

Chapter 10 - I *Hope* One Day: A Cure for Breast Cancer

Another charity close to my heart is **Breast Cancer UK,** *and its aim is to help prevent women and men developing breast cancer. The organisation uses the latest academic research on breast cancer prevention to provide guidance on how to reduce the risk.*

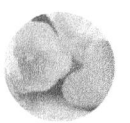

Breast Cancer Prevention

It is a fact that Breast Cancer is the most commonly diagnosed cancer in the UK. It is a fact that one in seven women will be diagnosed with breast cancer in their lifetime. But the good news is that over a quarter of breast cancer cases are preventable and if precautionary measures are adopted for a healthier lifestyle, the risk of developing breast cancer can be significantly reduced. From research, not everyone will go through the heavy treatments of chemotherapy. Unfortunately, when I was diagnosed, the cancer had spread and to prevent a worst-case scenario my first treatment was chemotherapy. It is important to stress that if you or a loved one is/has been faced with a breast cancer diagnosis it does not mean it was your fault! Personally, I experienced annoying aches under my armpit, which I ignored, because I was not aware that an ache under my armpit was also a symptom of breast cancer and I assumed it was muscular pains, due to muscle strengthening exercises. If there are any lumps in the breast, under the arms, itching, or discharge from the nipples, or any other abnormal changes in the breast or nipple, these are known to be the main symptoms. Although I have always made sure to keep an eye on my health, as far as I was concerned, I failed to take proper care. I felt I should have acted

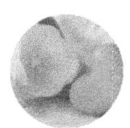

earlier, due to the pain and lump(s) appearing under my arm. Though, I would have panicked and without hesitation, made an emergency appointment with my GP.

Being diagnosed with breast cancer is a huge stressor and I had to encourage myself to eliminate blame or feel sorry for myself by maintaining a healthy and positive outlook. My journey encouraged me to undertake research to find relevant breast cancer websites and read books to become more knowledgeable about the type of breast cancer I was diagnosed with and how I could help myself and others. I now know, being aware is crucial for our survival and it was important to acknowledge any health issues/concerns. Therefore, we must take charge of our health and wellbeing and be persistent when taking charge and seeking professional guidance.

Breast Cancer UK Prevention – Reduce Your Risk

Physical Activity and Exercise

By being physically active, you can reduce your risk of breast cancer by around 20%. Physical activity reduces the risk of breast cancer recurrence and mortality, following a breast cancer diagnosis. It helps to lower the levels of certain circulating hormones and reduces inflammation that can help lower the likelihood of cancer developing and progressing. Physical activity, including structured exercise,

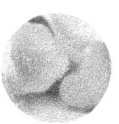

lowers levels of hormones such as oestrogen, androgen, insulin, leptin (a hormone associated with hunger) and certain growth factors. Increased levels of all of these have been associated with breast cancer. Being active also generally improves the capacity of the immune system to protect you from cancer. It keeps your weight under control that plays a significant role in lowering breast cancer risk, in women, who have reached menopause and in men. One study found as little as an hour of walking per week helps improve survival rates if you have breast cancer. Benefits were found in women who walked for 3–5 hours per week. There are a number of other factors to consider to help reduce the risk:

- Lifestyle changes
- Air Pollution & Pesticides
- Plastics
- Cleaning Products
- Cosmetics & Beauty Products

To learn more about breast cancer prevention and how we can reduce the risk of a breast cancer diagnosis, please visit:

https://www.breastcanceruk.org.uk

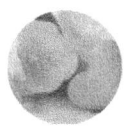

Chapter 11 - My Experience on Surviving

The **worst** *part about enduring cancer is that you see each day as a* **pain**. *Yet, the* **best** *part of surviving is when you start treating each day as a* **blessing**.

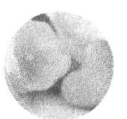

Cynthia Langdon

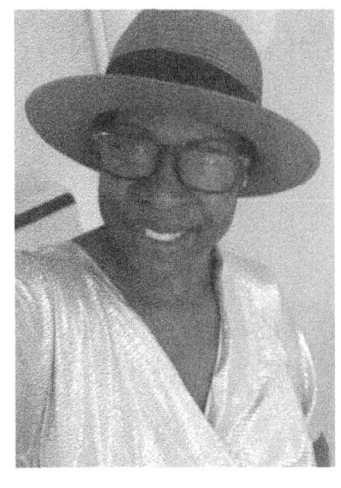

Why was being diagnosed with breast cancer became my blessing?

Surviving breast cancer provided me with growth and enlightenment and many unexpected and new opportunities. Surviving gave me a new lease of life, to focus on thriving and making significant life changes, such as pursuing my dreams, goals, being more mindful of my health, choosing closeness with those who make me feel good about myself, the importance of embracing each day and working on myself; by understanding what brings me joy. Each challenge we face can either change us or we can let it define us. Having been diagnosed with breast cancer taught me new things. Cancer is nasty, it is time-consuming and life changing but it gave me the chance to reflect on life and change something for a better future. I did have some precious moments being part of the community of fighters and survivors where we gave each other unconditional strength and support, and this is the most incredible community to be a part of.

I realised that I was loved, people cared, were kind and wanted to help and support me. Now and forever, I will always remember those

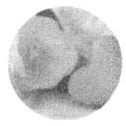

who stood by my bedside when I was struggling with chemotherapy. These people: families, friends, and acquaintances, despite having their own lives to live and families to care for, showed me unconditional kindness and support. Due to privacy, they will remain nameless, but they know who they are.

Life, before the breast cancer diagnosis, was pretty busy; working a full-time job, social commitments, daily activities, and networking events. I also enjoyed challenges and found myself taking on many projects, whether it was to help the community or myself. Some became overwhelming and this is something I now believe, also played a part in my illness. It is about focusing on one task at a time since subconsciously, I was burnt out and stressed because the mission had to be accomplished at all costs. Before my cancer diagnosis days, I found it difficult to say no. Today, my life missions are now my priorities, and these give meaning and happiness. First and foremost, to me – it is about self-care and investing in activities and habits that nurture my body and mind. My physical health is on top of my list of priorities.

Also at the top, is cultivating healthy relationships and spending quality time with my loved ones. Since they are my first pillar of support, I believe it is important to be surrounded by positivity and

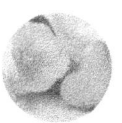

by people who will support and help me grow; make me feel better and make me laugh. Laughter is a great therapy for healing.

What Has My Diagnosis Taught Me?

Even as an independent person I also needed help, support, love and care. There were plans I made on how I wanted my life to be before my diagnosis. But it taught me how to receive love, help, and support from those who wanted to give. It also taught me how to ask for help. Before my diagnosis I probably did not appreciate life as I do today. The diagnosis taught me life is about adventures, taking risks and embracing new things. Since then, I have built my travel business and flown first class with British Airways, an awesome and comfortable experience. I have also written my first book, became a model and supporting artist for TV Films and commercials, and met a lot of inspiring and motivational people.

Being diagnosed with breast cancer makes one want to live life to the fullest because you realise that you are valuable, worthy and life is precious. We are here for a purpose and our time is limited. I am now not just surviving, I am thriving. I now have a new appreciation for life. I am kinder and more patient with myself and others. I know what it is like to be in a dark place and my mission is to spread the energy of positive thoughts and healing and acting as a role model, for those who may be struggling with a breast cancer diagnosis.

How has my life changed for the better?

I became more upbeat by having feelings of hope and telling myself every single day that *„I am doing well, and the future will be bright"*. This helped me during the challenges I faced as it was important for me to turn my negative emotions into positive ones since I was determined to survive. I was not going to be beaten by a breast cancer diagnosis as there was work to do! Going through my own experience I am now committed to supporting, helping, and caring for others, who may face the same or similar trials like myself, by helping to prevent and raise awareness. Although the treatments helped, they were debilitating and even though I got through them feeling stronger. I became clearer on my life priorities and my relationships; I appreciated the little things and value life even more.

How I created, a Breast Cancer Diagnosis Survivorship Plan, For My Health and Wellbeing

My Oncologist, Dr. Quigley, made me aware that surviving breast cancer began with the diagnosis and not after the treatment ended. A survivorship plan not only helped me to focus on my overall health and well-being but also my financial stability and emotional health. I

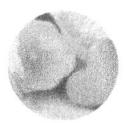

was encouraged by Dr. Quigley and the care team to follow established guidelines for good health. Since, after-treatment care was just as important as during treatment care, especially for survivors. They helped me to prepare and face the physical and emotional challenges of survivorship. I admit I had fears of the cancer returning. However, by creating this plan, it acted as my guide and reference, taking immediate action if I noticed anything abnormal. Furthermore, this plan acted as a reference if ever I needed to see a healthcare professional for anything else.

The plan included:

- The recording of my diagnosis and treatment history.

- The recording of any signs or side effects and symptoms.

- Listing my lifestyle, healthy eating habits and wellness changes.

- Increased exercise and physical activity.

- A strict record-keeping of all my appointments.

- Routine follow-ups of doctor and hospital visits for mammograms, bone density tests and so on.

- A comprehensive record of my test results.

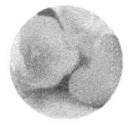

- Taking better care of myself.

- Ensuring I was rewarding myself.

- Ensuring I participated in clinical trials for survivors, such as testing for new cancer drugs. Including any side effects (I took part in the new Herceptin trial, which provided me with the opportunity to help others).

- I found books to be immensely helpful and a book I turned to was *"THE ULTIMATE GUIDE to Breast Cancer: Find Help, Hope and Healing"* by Mary L Gemignani MD, MPH with Caren Goldman. I also read several booklets, such as: *"Your Breasts, Your Health: throughout your life"*, *"A Practical Guide Living with and After Cancer"*, *"Moving Forward"* resources, available from Breast Cancer Now. Being aware about breast cancer increases the awareness and the information was important for healing, recovery and prevention.

What Further Self-Help I Did To Overcome My Challenges?

Finding my people

Beyond my immediate circle I found great comfort in sharing my experiences with people, even strangers, going through similar challenges. These people came from support groups I attended that

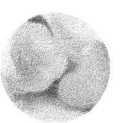

were organised by Breast Cancer Now. One of my fears was recurrence of breast cancer and I knew that I had to prevent this happening to me, by gaining knowledge of the risks. Lifestyle changes were the answer for me. Regular exercise, a change of food and spiritual belief. I also attended support groups that focused on emotional support. Both groups played an important role in my healing process, after my breast cancer diagnosis. It encouraged me to share my feelings with people, who may not necessarily have had the same type of breast cancer but as we were all under the same umbrella, it made it easier for us to understand and empathise. Not everyone will feel comfortable in attending support groups, asking questions or sharing their experiences with strangers. But I found meeting with these people was a powerful source of support and, to this day, I am still actively involved with these beautiful support groups. These groups provided complementary and holistic treatments and I enjoyed the complementary Reiki and yoga sessions.

The Power of Journaling

I had been journaling for years, it had been my source of spiritual support and before my cancer challenges, I had learnt a feeling of gratitude when I opened my eyes in the morning and wrote down

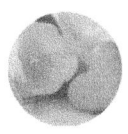

one positive thing before going to bed which was good for my mental health. Journaling helped me to not only survive but also to thrive. It was a way of caring for myself by recording daily events, making it easier to understand my thoughts, feelings, and experiences. A way to calm my anxiety and help combat any stress. My notes also helped my doctors and care team monitor my progress. It was not just about how I was feeling; it was also about how others made me feel and how grateful I was. I have come to believe journaling helped me to stay motivated and keep control of my emotions, even in my dark days. It became an active part of my healing process. This writing gave me the opportunity to process my emotions in a safe, contained space. It helped to reduce my tension, anxiety and stress, and boost my wellbeing. Journaling helped me to get to know myself and what I needed.

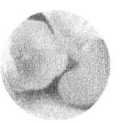

Cynthia Langdon

Chapter 12 - My Special Messages to You

To all my sisters and brothers who may be dealing with or watching a loved one deal with a breast cancer diagnosis, other cancers or severe illnesses.

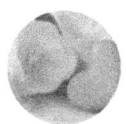

Find Your Inner Warrior – Your Own Uniqueness

I see you and I honour your journey. I hope these tips, gathered from my own experience, surviving and thriving, with a cancer diagnosis, will serve as guideposts on your path. You are warrior goddesses and gods, every one of you.

Sharing some Inspirational messages from the Breast Cancer Bosom Buddies:

Fighting cancer is a battle that is not won just by medicines, chemotherapy, and a wonderful team of doctors. Becoming cancer free also requires a constant stream of strong will power, faith, hope, love and most importantly, a cheerful outlook.

1. Cancer is not just a word; it is a language altogether. Cancer is not just about recovery by medicines; it is about healing yourself, from within.

2. Finding out that you are cancer-free can sometimes be more difficult to accept than finding out that you have cancer. Use this sense of disbelief to rid yourself of all the negative emotions and negative people.

3. Cancer is a disease that shows you how you cannot completely control how healthy you are. But recovery from

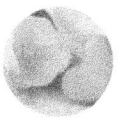

cancer will show you how you can completely control how happy you are.

4. Surviving cancer means that you will now constantly seek HAPPINESS, feel GRATITUDE, and spread LOVE.

5. Before cancer: love your job, laugh with your colleagues, be focused and do all the things you have been asked to do. After cancer: love your family, laugh with your friends, be positive and do all the things you have always wanted to do.

6. A wonderful team of doctors and medicines are just a part of the recovery. What matters more is the will power and desperation to kick the disease out of your body.

7. Cancer is life-threatening but recovery from it is life changing. The same chemotherapy, that once ruined your life, will now give you a fresh, new perspective to life. You will have different priorities, but one thing will always remain constant – the will to live.

8. It can be scary to learn that someone you love and care about has a breast cancer diagnosis. You may feel sad or worried and wonder how you can help them get through it.

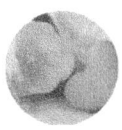

9. Be prepared for changes in your loved one's behaviour and mood. Medications and stress may make them feel depressed, angry, or tired.

10. Encourage them to be active and to do as much for themselves as possible. It will help them feel a sense of control.

11. How I accepted that I had a cancer diagnosis:

- Practiced ways to relax.
- Shared feelings honestly with family, friends, a spiritual advisor/counsellor.
- Keeping a journal to organise my thoughts.
- When faced with a difficult decision, listed the advantages and disadvantages for each choice.
- Found a source of spiritual support.

Sharing a final message, from my breast cancer bosom buddy, who supported me during, after and now – *Sharon Bashford*

"To be told you have cancer can never prepare you for the journey ahead and when Cynthia told me she did not want to undergo treatment, I began to explain my own cancer journey, at the time of

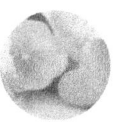

my own diagnosis, in March 2011. I had two young girls who relied on me, so to give up was out of the question. While my family was feeling emotionally distraught at the news, I was the one being positive and I remember thinking at the time, how dare they be upset when it was me who had cancer? I was the one who was going to be sick for the next six months.

I remained positive throughout my journey since I needed to continue with my routines, like taking the kids to school and go to work, while accepting I was going to be sick one week out of three as my treatment began. To be feeling okayish for two weeks out of three, kept me focused. So, for Cynthia to tell me she was refusing treatment I knew I wanted to explain to her that by remaining positive it would see her through. Yes, she would still get sick and yes, she would lose her hair but hair grows back!!

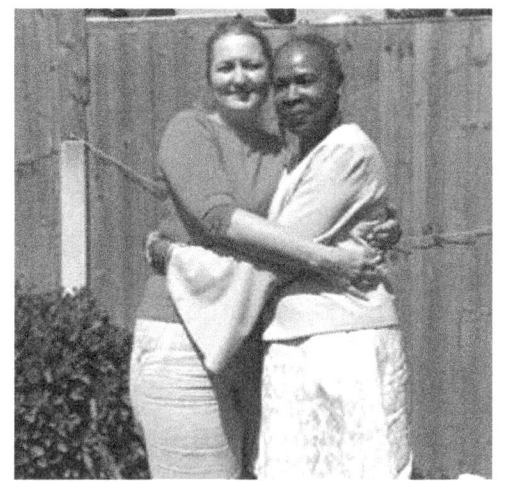

Having gone through a life-threatening illness such as cancer, it makes one appreciate the little things in life even more It is so

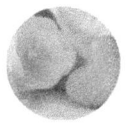

precious and whether you like it or not, it forces you to re-evaluate how you live it. I will be cancer free for ten years in March 2022. Having gone through our cancer journey I have gained a special friend in Cynthia, who to this day, remains upbeat and positive. You are truly an inspirational woman. XXX"

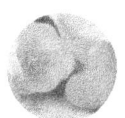

Preface

"A joyful heart is a good medicine – A cheerful heart brings good healing"

Proverbs 17:22

"You try so hard to go back to that person you were, but **you are somebody new**. *The sooner you embrace who you've become; you welcome everyone else to do so."*

Breast Cancer Changes You, and The Change Can Be Beautiful.

This book is a gift to me and a special gift to the world. Being diagnosed with breast cancer changed my life dramatically. Everyone, who goes through breast cancer, has their own story to tell. My story is a celebratory gift to myself of overcoming fear, isolation, mental and physical emotions, to embracing and living the most beautiful life.

My aim!

A Breast cancer diagnosis impacts the lives of so many, and it is important to bring attention to it and help support, finding a cure and getting involved, in raising awareness and sharing information.

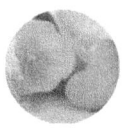

Acknowledgements

I would like to say a huge thank you, to all my friends and family who have shown kindness and generosity along the way. You have been a power of strength and have supported me, by being there for me, when I needed it most. You all enriched my life more than you will ever know. My heartfelt appreciation, love and gratitude to you.

A special thank you, to **Mauray Jacobie**, for his dedicated kindness, care, positivity, unconditional love and support during this season. Words alone, cannot express my sincere love and thankfulness to all the family. Forever grateful.

My brother – **Clarence Langdon,** for his input and words of encouragement.

Gill Tiney, for her encouragement in getting me started to write and share my story to the world.

Kwame M A McPherson, my book mentor and editor, for his patience and who supported and trusted me enough to know it had to be done.

My Bosom Model Buddies (BMB) of October 2016 been through a breast cancer diagnosis, we were all able to discuss our experiences with confidence and be cheerful. My BMB continued to

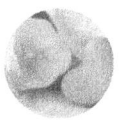

uplift my spirits, supported, motivated, and inspired me to get this book written.

My dear school friend – **Terence Thomas** for his continued support.

Recognition

Heartfelt appreciation and humble recognition are given for permissions granted by the following charity organisations:

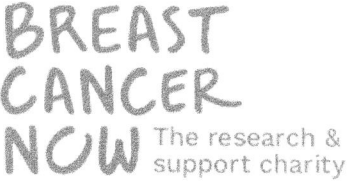

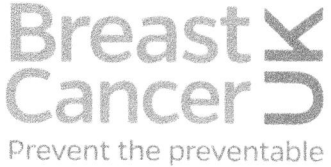

Charities make so much difference to the lives of cancer sufferers and to the lives of their friends, family, and carers.

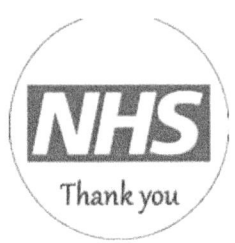

I want to take this time to say how grateful I am for the wonderful healthcare team at Queens and Bart's hospitals. Everyone who helped and cared for me. The Registrars, Nurses, and other remarkable hospital staff. Dr. Mary Quigley (Oncologist), Mr. Ojo (Surgeon), Sunflower Ward, Psychotherapist, Physiotherapist, and Massage Therapists for providing the care and attention I needed, to get me through this season.

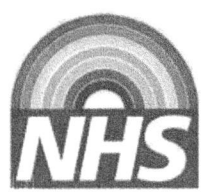

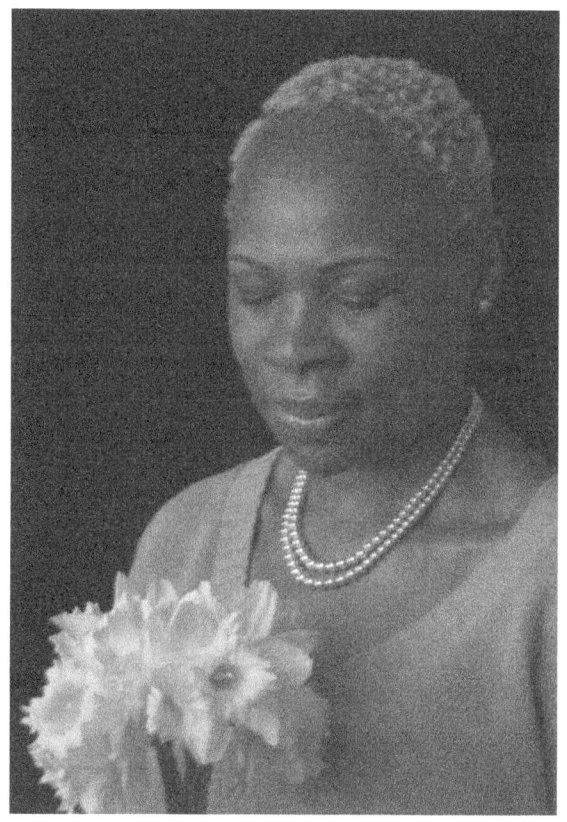

Thank you to Roy Wilson for my book cover photos

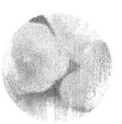

Cynthia Langdon

When you purchase this book 4% will be donated to Breast Cancer Now and Breast Cancer UK

THANK YOU!

Cynthia